'A central pillar of the psychoanalytic vision of human experience, often overlooked in favor of themes that attract more popular attention, is how each of us deals with the losses that inevitably accompany growth at every step in development. These losses, of the relationships that taught us to love and of our own omnipotent power to create them, must be mourned if we are to be able to live freely and effectively. This understanding, first suggested by Freud and later elaborated in the work of Melanie Klein, Hans Loewald, and others, remains incomplete. In this volume, John Steiner brilliantly and movingly continues the conversation. It is essential reading for anybody interested in appreciating the best that psychoanalysis has to offer.'

Jay Greenberg, *PhD, faculty, William Alanson White Institute, former editor,* The Psychoanalytic Quarterly, *recipient, 2015 Mary S. Sigourney Award*

'In this impressive and illuminating work, John Steiner covers a wide range of topics with great insight and intelligence. His exploration of the processes involved in mourning are particularly useful, important and original, but the book also contains fascinating chapters in which he uses references to the work of Shakespeare or Homer to illustrate and enrich his psychoanalytic insights.'

Michael Feldman, *training analyst, British Psychoanalytical Society*

'This book has a lustrous quality. It is simply the best written on its topic.

With unrivaled experience and remarkable breadth and depth of sensibility, knowledge and intellectual capacity, Steiner builds his framework joining the insights of Freud and Melanie Klein with those of World Literature.

With this, step by step, Steiner guides his reader through what is one of the hardest tasks of the human condition… the need to grieve if we are to recover truly from our losses, yet the great difficulty of what this involves.

Steiner identifies the gaps in our understanding of what is involved. He endorses the necessity of protest against the senses of injury and injustice. As he writes, a quiet, profound sense of humanity is revealed.'

David Taylor, *psychoanalyst, Visiting Professor UCL Psychoanalysis Unit*

Explorations of Mourning in Psychoanalysis and Literature

This book explores the conflict between holding on to and letting go of loss, paying homage to Freud's classic 'Mourning and Melancholia' and building on its foundation with contemporary ideas.

Losses are met throughout life and are either accepted and mourned or resented and denied. Sometimes mourning is inappropriate or premature because losses can be prevented, and unfinished business needs to be completed. Eventually, however, accepting and mourning the loss confers enormous benefits, many of which arise from the development of symbolic thinking that enables ghosts to be turned into ancestors. These themes are explored in clinical material and in extracts from literature. They enable some of the ideas of Freud, Klein, and Bion to be expanded and updated. The book ends with an edited transcript of interviews discussing the author's personal history in relation to his work.

With insights from across the author's distinguished psychoanalytic career and a deep understanding of literature, this is key reading for all psychoanalysts, and anyone who wants to understand loss.

John Steiner is a training analyst of the British Psychoanalytical Society. He was formerly a psychiatrist at the Maudsley Hospital and a psychotherapist at the Tavistock Clinic. He is now retired from clinical practice but continues to supervise and write. He is the author of *Psychic Retreats* (1993), *Seeing and Being Seen* (2011), and *Illusion, Disillusion, and Irony in Psychoanalysis* (2020). He has also edited and written introductions to *The Oedipus Complex Today* (1989), *Psychoanalysis, Literature and War* (1997), *Rosenfeld in Retrospect* (2008), and *Lectures on Technique by Melanie Klein* (2017).

Explorations of Mourning in Psychoanalysis and Literature

Turning Ghosts into Ancestors

John Steiner

Routledge
Taylor & Francis Group
LONDON AND NEW YORK

Designed cover image: © Nick Garland

First published 2026
by Routledge
4 Park Square, Milton Park, Abingdon, Oxon OX14 4RN

and by Routledge
605 Third Avenue, New York, NY 10158

Routledge is an imprint of the Taylor & Francis Group, an informa business

British Library Cataloguing-in-Publication Data
A catalogue record for this book is available from the British Library

ISBN: 9781041212195 (hbk)
ISBN: 9781041201199 (pbk)
ISBN: 9781003726135 (ebk)

DOI: 10.4324/9781003726135

Typeset in Optima
by codeMantra

To the memory of Ignês Sodré and Ron Britton.

Contents

Acknowledgements

I would like to thank the many people who have helped to get this book produced. Of course, most of all my wife Deborah, to whom I have read all of the chapters as the various versions were adapted with her patient help and comments.

All of the chapters have been, in one form or another, presented at the annual West Lodge conferences conducted for many years by Michael Feldman, Ron Britton, Priscilla Roth, and me.

It is sad to have to acknowledge the loss of Ron Britton and also of Ignês Sodré, both of whom died in 2025 and both of whom were a huge influence on my work.

My colleague Heinz Weiss, who kindly wrote the preface, has also discussed my work regularly for many years.

I would also like to thank Nick Garland, whose painting from Hampstead Heath was commissioned to serve as the book cover.

Although I have not seen analytic patients for several years now, I have kept in touch with clinical material through supervision and seminars where the themes in this book have been explored. Nina Varchevker and Elaine Reinertsen provided the clinical material for one of the papers, and Elaine was of tremendous help in the editing and revision of the whole book. To all of them I am deeply grateful.

Preface

Heinz Weiss

'Turning ghosts into ancestors' deals with a universal human condition: the acceptance of mourning and loss, and therefore the acknowledgement of time.

John Steiner's new book is not only a brilliant exposé of his research into the process of mourning over almost four decades, it also offers a new and often surprising slant into the pain and obstacles which make mourning so difficult. The starting point is Freud's paper on 'Mourning and Melancholia' (Freud, 1917b), as well as Melanie Klein's (1940, 1946) seminal work on the transition from the paranoid-schizoid to depressive states of mind that makes mourning possible.

Ghosts cannot be mourned but only defeated. Ancestors, however, must be mourned so as to remain alive in our memory. As the author explains, this process is painful and difficult, but allows us to leave the past behind and to open ourselves up to new experiences.

In his 1993 book *Psychic Retreats* (Steiner, 1993a), Steiner differentiated between the *fear of loss* and the *experience of loss*, arguing that split-off parts of the self which have been projected into the object must be regained so as to experience *separateness*. And it is precisely here where mourning sets in. In this new work, the author speaks of the *turning point of mourning*, which is essential for the decision to let the object go or to hold on to it through omnipotent illusions, narcissistic identifications, or grievances, which all operate as powerful obstacles against mourning.

The whole book can be read as an outstanding and subtle analysis of these processes, be it in literature or in the clinical situation. John Steiner's profound clinical experience with narcissistic, borderline, and psychotic patients gives him a deep insight into those obstacles which prevail in what he has come to call 'pathological organisations of the personality'.

Of course, mourning is painful, and we often resist and rebel against it. But, finally, we must be able to relinquish our objects so as to give them a place in our memory. Or, to put it into the words of Roger Money-Kyrle, one of Steiner's theoretical 'ancestors': 'Without the memory there can be no mourning, and without the mourning there can be no memory' (Money-Kyrle, 1971, p. 444).

John Steiner's new ideas can be seen as an exploration in depth of this complex interdependency.

Another important turning point is *the transition from concrete to symbolic thinking*. As the author makes clear, both forms of thought coexist throughout our lives. In order to be receptive to the patient's concrete communications, the analyst's capacity to take them in is an important step before he becomes able to transform them though creative imagination. This again is a prerequisite for re-projecting them in a more digestible form into the patient.

This process has been described as 'reparation' (Money-Kyrle, 1971) or as maternal reverie (Bion, 1962). John Steiner adds here an important point: *the interplay between 'horizontal' and 'vertical' ways of communication*, which represent two different forms of relationship. Whereas the *horizontal communication* may be compared to the relation between the baby's mouth and the mother's breast, the *vertical communication* represents an up-and-down relationship, like the relation between mind and bottom. Whilst the first type may give rise to narcissistic illusions, like the phantasy of the Garden of Eden, the second represents a struggle over power and domination. Both can turn into each other like a seesaw.

The problem is that most human relationships, like the relation between parents and child or the relation between patient and analyst, are at the same time *reciprocal* and *asymmetric*. If the longing for power prevails, it gives rise to grievance, humiliation, and shame, which operate as powerful obstacles against mourning. As Steiner hints, receptiveness and the longing to exert control over the object are incompatible with each other. The equilibrium between freedom and order in the analytic session, which includes the necessity for the patient's consent for the boundaries of the setting, is examined in a special chapter.

John Steiner has dealt with these themes before in previous publications, like 'The Conflict between Mourning and Melancholia' (Steiner, 2005) or 'The Struggle for Dominance in the Oedipus Situation' (Steiner, 1999). But they are now deepened and brought together in a consistent theory. As he makes clear in his reflection on Freud's (1923) seminal paper 'The Ego and the Id', the up-and-down relationship also accounts for the super-ego's relation with the ego. He argues that it might be necessary for the ego to stand up against the primitive figures which prevail in the deep unconscious and can hardly be modified.

Examples from classical literature, like Achilles' wrath in Homer's *Iliad*; the role of the gaze in romantic relationships, as expressed in Shakespeare's three caskets in *The Merchant of Venice*; or Hamlet's longing for revenge, constitute an important part of the book. They are not only revealing for the study of literature, but also for the practising analyst.

Referring to new material from the Klein Archives (Steiner, 2017; English, 2023) Steiner revisits Klein's theory of mourning. The chapters on the 'impostor' and the development of a personal identity are closely connected to his postgraduate seminar, which is a unique source of creativity.

Concluding the book is an interview with Daniel Pick, which gives insight into Steiner's work and life.

In my view, the twelve chapters of John Steiner's new book offer a brilliant and new integration of the ideas he has developed over the last ten years. It will be required reading not only for the practising analyst, but for all those who are preoccupied with the peculiarities of mourning, like writers, artists, social workers, philosophers, historians, and other scientists.

Introduction

> Those who know ghosts tell us that they long to be released from their ghost life and led to rest as ancestors.
>
> (Loewald,1960, p. 248)

I owe the title of this book to Hans Loewald (1906–1993), a highly respected American psychoanalyst who described internal objects that can haunt us like ghosts and block development unless they can be transformed into ancestors. Psychoanalysts are familiar with such ghosts, which arise when lost objects have not been fully mourned. They are set up as internal objects that haunt the subject in the present, and the essence of the analytic task is often to enable the work of mourning in order to relegate them to the past as ancestors.

Introduction and Outline

The turning of ghosts into ancestors is a central theme of this book. In it, I argue that the essence of the change involves the transformation of a concrete internal object into its symbolic counterpart. As a symbol, the lost object continues to exert an influence, but its status has changed. It has been transformed from a concrete object making concrete demands into a figure that can appear in memories, phantasies and dreams, where its demands become symbolic and hence less onerous. In this way it remains important, but as an ancestor. While our understanding of this transformation is far from complete, the outcome has a substantial effect on development and marks the difference between the limitations of concrete thinking and the freedom achieved when symbolic thinking is possible.

Mourning certainly plays a critical part, and the understanding of the factors that facilitate or obstruct mourning will occupy much of the book. The extraordinary insight of Freud's 'Mourning and Melancholia' (1917b) remains the definitive account, and allows us to see how mourning can liberate the personality when successful and leave the patient trapped in melancholia when it fails.

DOI: 10.4324/9781003726135-1

The Discovery of the Internal World

Freud showed that after a loss the external object was replaced by an internal counterpart, retained through internalisation and identification. This realisation enabled Freud to look inward and discover a rich internal world containing objects in a relationship with the self and with each other. It allowed psychoanalysis to shift attention away from its preoccupation with infantile trauma, which was now recognised as interacting with objects in the internal world. Once it was envisaged, the internal world enabled Freud to develop a structural model of the mind based on the relationship between id, ego, and super-ego (1923), which became the foundation of contemporary object relations theories (Klein,1952; Winnicott, 1965; Ogden, 2002).

The Character of the Ego

While the lost object primarily affects the character of the super-ego, Freud saw that the ego is also profoundly affected by the manner in which the losses of life are negotiated.

> When it happens that a person has to give up a sexual object, there quite often ensues an alteration of his ego which can only be described as a setting up of the object inside the ego, as it occurs in melancholia; ... It may be that this identification is the sole condition under which the id can give up its objects. At any rate the process, especially in the early phases of development, is a very frequent one, and it makes it possible to suppose that the character of the ego is a precipitate of abandoned object-cathexes and that it contains the history of those object-choices. (Freud, 1923, p. 29)

I think Freud implies that both the ego and super-ego are influenced when the lost object is set up internally. When it is retained through identification, it takes on the character of the super-ego in melancholia. When it can be relinquished and mourned it becomes an *abandoned* object, as libido is withdrawn and affects the ego as an ancestor. We gain our identity and character from identification with our lost objects, but a true personal identity requires a dis-identification between self and object. All of this points to the importance of mourning throughout life, because a failure to separate and mourn leaves us at the mercy of ghosts, over-identified with our objects and without a mind of our own.

Accepting or Denying Loss

It is clear that mourning is important from the beginning of life because every developmental step involves letting go of the old and embracing the new. This means that the pain of loss must be faced in the ordinary separations of weaning, sleeping separately, leaving home, and eventually facing the inevitable losses of death. Each of the changes may be resisted as unjust and each may revive early wounds that make the loss difficult to accept.

The Turning Point of Mourning

It is this conflict between acceptance and rebellion that appears in response to every loss and determines whether the mourner moves on to new developments or stays trapped in old relationships. The choice can be so difficult and the consequences so important that I refer to the point of change as the *turning point of mourning.* Rebelling against the injustice of the loss, and fighting to put right the injury, are not always wrong, and it is important to recognise that sometimes losses can be delayed, prevented, or reversed.

In melancholia the internalised object acquires a judgemental super-ego role, and its injunctions and commands are commonly resented but cannot be ignored. Moreover when its demands are experienced concretely, they are felt to be beyond the patient's ordinary means and in these circumstances, omnipotent phantasies may be turned to. Omnipotence plays a critical role when it is used to preserve the object and make mourning unnecessary and is one of the factors that determines how we cope with loss. There are times when omnipotence is useful in the struggle against loss, but eventually it must be relinquished, and omnipotence itself has to be mourned if development is to proceed.

The Work of Mourning

Freud described how in the work of mourning every memory and expectation of the lost object must be examined and the verdict of reality applied. This verdict says either that the object is dead and must be mourned, or that it can be kept alive either externally or as a ghost in the internal world. If it can be mourned, libido is withdrawn from it and the self and object are allowed to be seen as separate. If it is left to reside as a ghost, the result is melancholia, with its burdens of concrete thinking.

While Freud's account remains unchallenged as the basic model of mourning, our understanding is enhanced if we expand our thinking to include contemporary views. For me, Klein's account of splitting and projective identification is especially important because it enables us to recognise that Freud's lost internalised object is a *composite-object,* a term I use to emphasise that the object has been altered through the projection into it of elements of the self. Its composite nature means that the self relates, not to a separate object, but to the self in the object, and projective identification can be thought to underlie the narcissistic object relationship which Freud postulated was a prerequisite of melancholia.

The composite nature of the lost object enables us to specify more precisely what comprises the work of mourning. Freud (1917b) described it as involving the withdrawal of libido from the lost object so that it can be returned to the self, eventually to be invested in new objects. A central theme developed throughout this book is the idea that, in addition to libido, parts of the self that have been projected into the object must also be withdrawn if mourning is to be successful. This is not a new idea. In her influential paper on symbol formation, Segal (1957) proposed that concrete objects are created through projective identification and that symbolic function requires self and object to be seen as separate.

The withdrawal of such projections can be felt as a painful tearing away, and it is not surprising that it is dreaded and avoided. Yet it is an essential aspect of the mourning process (Steiner, 1993b, pp. 54–63), and is so critical for development that it can be thought of as an important aim of psychoanalytic therapy. Rather than helping them to negotiate the conflicts of life, the analysis can help the patient regain elements of themselves that enhance their resources so that they can deal with their conflicts themselves (Steiner, 1996a).

When we recognise that separating from the object involves not just a withdrawal of libido and includes separating elements of the self, we can see that the task is complex, and much depends on the success of the work. If the withdrawal is effective the patient feels more free, both self and object are less distorted, and the concrete thinking becomes symbolic. If they cannot withdraw the projections, the patient is left in a melancholic state at the mercy of concrete composite-objects.

Factors that Block Mourning

Another prominent theme in the book is the need to understand the factors that block mourning and prevent the turning point from being reached. Also, at times it is certainly necessary to delay mourning in order to work through problems in the relationship with the lost object. It may be premature to mourn while there is unfinished business to be concluded. Indeed, it may be that protest and rebellion have to be expressed and worked through before loss can be accepted and mourning can properly be embarked upon.

Outline of the Book

Chapter 1, 'Mourning and Melancholia: A Review and Kleinian Addendum', is devoted to a review of 'Mourning and Melancholia' (1917b), which is central to the book. It is here that I outline Klein's descriptions of splitting and projective identification, which allow us to recognise the internal object in melancholia as a composite-object and to view the work of mourning as involving not just the withdrawal of libido but also the withdrawal of the projected parts of the self.

In Chapter 2, 'Before and After the Fall: Horizontal and Vertical Object Orientations in the Analysis of a Patient with Grievances', the study of obstacles to mourning begins, with a description of the vertical relationship between ego and super-ego. This up-and-down relationship is inevitably contrasted with the idealised relationship between infant and mother, which is viewed as horizontal. It is when this idealised illusion is shattered that the fall from Paradise gives rise to the vertical relationship of mutual grievance that can block mourning. Clinical material is presented to illustrate the fact that mourning can sometimes be resumed if a softening of grievances can allow a degree of rapprochement to take place.

In Chapter 3, 'Mourning in Hamlet: Turning Ghosts into Ancestors', Loewald's idea of turning of ghosts into ancestors is illustrated by the ghost of Hamlet's father as an example of a concrete internalisation of a lost object. The ghost is installed as a severe super-ego making concrete demands for revenge and reparation. Hamlet's mourning for his dead father is blocked when the ghost fuels grievances provoked by his mother's over-hasty marriage. In his famous injunction, 'Remember me', the ghost occupies Hamlet's mind to the exclusion of all else and provokes violent phantasies towards others and himself. Gradually we see Hamlet detaching himself from his father's ghost, as he recognises that he does not share the chivalric values necessary for obedience as a son. Letting his father go enables the ghost to be returned to the grave and his father to be mourned and represented symbolically as an ancestor. The acceptance of the reality of loss ultimately includes the reality of Hamlet's own death.

In Chapter 4, 'Injury, Rage, Grievance, and Revenge in the Wrath of Achilles', the differences between grievance and revenge are explored in the wrath of Achilles in Homer's *Iliad*. Both arise in response to feelings of hurt and injustice, but revenge is expressed openly as a violent attack while grievance holds the violence inwardly in a state of withdrawal. This was the case with the rage of Achilles, which was initially expressed as a withdrawal and only later, following the death of his dear friend Patroclus, transformed into a violent rampage of revenge. It is argued that keeping and nursing a grudge internally makes it difficult to recognise its destructiveness, and expressing the grievance as revenge at least brings the violence out into the light of day. It may even be that externalising the rage in one form or another is an essential step in the recognition of the damage done and the reparation that is required.

In Chapter 5, 'Successful and Unsuccessful Mourning: Revisiting Klein', Klein's paper on mourning (1940) is used to illustrate how, in successful mourning, the self is able to be detached from the object which can then be recognised as lost. Klein describes how in a dream her patient, Mrs A, at first tried to follow her son as he fell to his death, but was able to pull herself away from the danger back to life. This was possible even though the revival of an early grievance against her idealised older brother led to hostility and triumph which blocked mourning for a while. The case is especially poignant if we accept that it is likely that Mrs A was a slightly disguised version of Klein herself. Klein considered her mourning to be successful, and contrasted it with the case of Mr B, who was unable to mourn because grievance, hostility and triumph were more deeply entrenched.

The discovery of new material about Mr B in the Klein Archives (Steiner, 2017; English, 2023) makes it possible to explore other factors that create obstacles to mourning. For example, the trauma and humiliation of being expelled from the nursery when his sister was born, when he was five, was revived when he bumped into another of Klein's patients. A difficult period of extreme hostility ensued in which Mr B expressed his hatred towards both the other patient and Klein herself, which she managed to endure. The analysis continued, and eventually some softening of the grievance allowed Mr B's sorrow and appreciation to emerge.

Chapter 6, 'To Modify or to Defy the Super-Ego: Revisiting "The Ego and the Id"', appeared in a volume of *The International Journal of Psychoanalysis* which commemorated one hundred years since the publication of 'The Ego and the Id' (Freud, 1923). Klein was enormously influenced by Freud's paper, which codified the findings from 'Mourning and Melancholia' (Freud, 1917b) and established a structural theory of the mind. It confirms the super-ego as an internal object that looks down on the ego, making judgements on it and, in melancholia, becoming pathologically severe. Klein was amply to confirm its punitive nature in many of her child patients, and she saw one of the aims of analysis being to modify its severity.

However, Klein also recognised that it was not always possible to tame the savagery of the super-ego, which seemed to exist unchanged as a primitive figure in the deep unconscious. In these cases, rather than modifying the super-ego it may be necessary to stand up to it. Here Britton's idea of emancipating the ego from the dominance of the super-ego becomes important (Britton, 2018). It is especially the ego's right to make judgements that needs to be reclaimed, and this includes judging the super-ego itself.

Chapter 7, 'Romantic and Mature Love: "Tell me where is fancy bred"', is focussed on a remarkable poem that appears in the three-caskets scene of Shakespeare's *The Merchant of Venice*. It asks, 'Where is fancy bred?' and concludes that it is bred not in the heart or head but in the eyes. It is through the gaze that the romance is engendered and creates an excited attachment based on appearance. The poem suggests that it is through confronting death that romantic love can mature into a deeper kind of loving.

Other scenes from the play are used to explore the importance of suffering, and mourning the loss of the ideal, in order to cement the romantic relationship into something more real. Perhaps it is the adoption of an ironic stance that makes the loss of the ideal more bearable, since it permits the pleasures of romance without believing them to be literally true.

Chapter 8, 'Chaos, Freedom, and Order in the Analytic Setting', describes how the analyst attempts to create a setting in which freedom of thought for both patient and analyst are protected from unchecked chaos on the one hand and excessive order on the other. The function of containment, so essential in the handling of anxiety, can fail if the mother is unable to receive the projections and give them meaning. If she creates a rigid order to protect herself from anxiety and chaos, the patient may internalise an exoskeleton that relieves anxiety at the expense of freedom. If this is relived in the analytic setting, the patient may feel that the analyst insists on rigid boundaries that are imposed without their consent. In a bid for freedom, they may need to rebel against such constraints, and to do this the maternal exoskeleton must be complemented with something like a paternal backbone that defends the freedom and safety of both the patient and the analyst.

The boundaries of the setting establish differences between patient and analyst that are difficult for the patient to accept, and of these the refusal to share personal information may be especially provocative. The freedom to rebel against these restrictions is an important right that can lead to a renegotiation to establish an order with consent rather than one based on authority. The struggle for freedom between patient and analyst can lead to a liberation of the ego from the tyranny of the super-ego.

Chapter 9, 'The Advantages and Disadvantages of Concrete Thinking: The Numbing Feeling of Reality', is based on an early paper on groups in which Bion (1961) described how the projection of concrete objects into the analyst is especially prone to take over the analyst's mind and paralyse the analyst's thinking. The patient may seem to be making a communication but is in fact evacuating a part of themselves in order to create a delusional idea that they need for their own equilibrium. If there is an excessive emphasis on reality in the clinical material, such delusional ideas become difficult to discern because they are presented as entirely reasonable. This means that the analyst fails to recognise that their mind is being taken over because it is blocked by the numbing effect of reality. I suggest that the numbing effect is enhanced when moral considerations support the patient's contention that their beliefs are entirely reasonable, and a double danger exists from the presence of both too much morality and too much reality.

Chapter 10, 'Acquiring a Personal Identity', is based on a short discussion of personal identity written as a foreword to a book on identity, which originated in my postgraduate workshop (Numa, 2023).[1] It differentiates a personal identity from the tribal identity we inherit from a family, school, nation, religion, profession, gender, or race. We introject the values of these 'ancestors', but in addition and sometimes in a reaction against these, we wish to forge an independent set of beliefs and values that help to answer the question 'Who am I?'

Applying the ideas on mourning discussed in other chapters, the ability to create a separate identity is linked to the capacity to let go of the internalised parents and mourn them.

In Chapter 11, 'The Impostor Revisited', the theme of personal identity is continued as the nature of the impostor is re-examined. This paper (Steiner,

1 This book was written by members of the workshop I have conducted over many years. Members presented clinical material and then discussed their papers as they were being prepared.

2011c) was commissioned to commemorate the classical accounts of Phyllis Greenacre and Helene Deutsch, each of which stresses how common it is to find impostors among our patients and colleagues, and also within ourselves.

We all seek admiration and external validation of our worth, and we may accuse ourselves that our identity is based on fraud, especially if we have failed to forge a secure personal identity that distinguishes ourselves from the beliefs and attitudes of others. Authenticity is an important ideal, but a residual suspicion of being an impostor may linger on.

Chapter 12, 'Personal Reminiscences from Interviews with Daniel Pick', is the final chapter of the book. It looks back at my early years and considers their influence on my interest in psychoanalysis. Daniel Pick skilfully made these links in several interviews, which cover many of the ideas developed throughout the book.

My views on the work of mourning, and the factors that facilitate or obstruct it, are described in several of the chapters. They are outlined in Chapter 1, and applied to the analysis of Mr D in Chapter 2. They are illustrated in the mourning of Shakespeare's *Hamlet* in Chapter 3, and Homer's Achilles in Chapter 4, in both of which grievance was a major inhibiting factor. Again, they are discussed in Chapter 5 in relation to Klein's patients, Mrs A and Mr B, from her paper on mourning, and in Chapter 6 are related to Freud's descriptions in *The Ego and The Id*. This makes for considerable repetition, but allows each of the chapters to be considered independently.

1 Mourning and Melancholia

A Review and Kleinian Addendum[1]

Introduction

Freud's 'Mourning and Melancholia' (1917b) plays such a central role in this book that it seems important to review its findings. Freud's fundamental discoveries showed how the work of mourning, when successful, can release the mourner to engage once more in life, and when obstructed, can lead to the development of melancholia. It is a sobering thought that more than a hundred years have passed since the publication of 'Mourning and Melancholia' without the need to make any substantial modification, and yet Klein's work, especially her description of projective identification, has enabled some of the mechanisms which underlie mourning to be clarified and added to.

Freud's sensitivity to the patient's suffering led him to understand the patient's need to hold on to the lost object through the mechanisms of internalisation and identification, and yet Freud could also recognise that eventually the reality of the loss had to be faced so that mourning could proceed. He began with a comparison of the two conditions and used his observations of melancholia to draw attention to the narcissistic nature of the object-relationship, which prevents the withdrawal of libido from the internalised lost object, as should happen in mourning. In this way the lost object becomes established internally, where it functions as an abnormal super-ego making demands on the ego. These observations by Freud, which I will elaborate later, have not been bettered in the intervening years.

Contemporary ideas have, however, filled in some of the gaps and have clarified some of the mechanisms. For me this is especially true of Klein's discovery of projective identification, which underlies the narcissistic object-relationship that Freud saw to be characteristic of melancholia. It is the projection of split-off parts of the self into the object that establishes it as a *composite-object*, and which allows us to see the work of mourning as involving not only the withdrawal of libido as Freud suggests but the withdrawal of these projections as well. I will proceed to survey Freud's account and update it from a contemporary Kleinian perspective where it seems appropriate.

1 This chapter has not previously been published.

DOI: 10.4324/9781003726135-2

Internalisation and Identification as Defence Against Loss

Freud saw that the experience of loss can be so shocking and so painful that the reality of the loss is denied through the object's becoming concretely established in the internal world, where it is related to as if it were still alive. The phantasy behind the internalisation is that of cannibalistic incorporation: 'The ego wants to incorporate this object into itself, and, in accordance with the oral or cannibalistic phase of libidinal development in which it is, it wants to do so by devouring it' (Freud, 1917b, p. 249). Freud had outlined this process in 'Totem and Taboo' (1913b) in the following way: 'One day the brothers who had been driven out came together, killed and devoured their father and so made an end of the patriarchal horde.... The dead father became stronger than the living one had been' (Freud, 1913b, pp. 141–143).

Unless mourning can be successfully concluded, it is this internalisation and identification that give rise to melancholia: 'In ... the painful disorder of melancholia ... an object which was lost has been set up again inside the ego – that is, that an object-cathexis has been replaced by an identification' (Freud, 1923, p. 28). He clarified this later, stating that

> A portion of the external world has, at least partially, been abandoned as an object and has instead, by identification, been taken into the ego and thus become an integral part of the internal world. This new psychical agency continues to carry on the functions which have hitherto been performed by the people [the abandoned objects] in the external world. (1940, p. 205)

However, in a significant later extension of his model Freud argued that this process of internalisation and identification was not limited to melancholia but was in fact a general response to loss.

> When it happens that a person has to give up a sexual object, there quite often ensues an alteration of his ego which can only be described as a setting up of the object inside the ego, as it occurs in melancholia; ... It may be that this identification is the sole condition under which the id can give up its objects. At any rate the process, especially in the early phases of development, is a very frequent one, and it makes it possible to suppose that the character of the ego is a precipitate of abandoned object-cathexes and that it contains the history of those object-choices. (Freud, 1923, p. 29)

In my view, Freud is suggesting that every loss is initially dealt with through an internalisation, indeed that a melancholic type of identification is necessary before the object can be relinquished. This means that even a normal mourning begins with a melancholic attachment through which the lost object is set up inside the ego. If mourning is successful, this object is eventually relinquished, while if it fails the object is retained and the result is melancholia.

Butler (1995) puts it well when she writes,

> For there is no final breaking of the attachment; there is, rather, the incorporation of the attachment as identification, where identification becomes a magical, a psychic, form of preserving the object. … the lost object continues to haunt and inhabit the ego as one of its constitutive identifications and … one might conclude that melancholic identification permits the loss of the object in the external world precisely because it provides a way to preserve the object as part of the ego itself and, hence, to avert the loss as a complete loss. Here we see that letting the object go means, paradoxically, that there is no full abandonment of the object, only a transferring of the status of the object from external to internal; giving up the object becomes possible only on condition of a melancholic internalization or, what might for our purposes turn out to be even more important, a melancholic incorporation. (Butler, 1995, p. 167)

Precisely the same internalisation takes place in mourning but is normally transitory, because as a result of the work of mourning the lost object is eventually let go and accepted as lost. I think it is important to note that even when relinquished, the lost object does not disappear from the internal world, but its status changes. It is de-cathected, libido is removed from it, so that it no longer possesses and haunts the mind as it is transformed from the world of concrete thinking to that of the symbolic. This transformation will be examined shortly, but first I will discuss the work of mourning, which Freud so meticulously described.

The Work of Mourning

Freud recognised that the work of mourning involves a separation between self and object, the self continuing to be alive and in the present, while the object has to be recognised as having died and existing in the past. It is because the object continues to exist internally as a concrete presence that the work of mourning is required to relegate it to the realm of memory and the imagination. Freud formulated this in terms of a withdrawal of libido that had become narcissistically fixed to the lost object and had to be detached from it. It is this demand that arouses opposition.

> Reality-testing has shown that the loved object no longer exists, and it proceeds to demand that all libido shall be withdrawn from its attachments to that object.
>
> This demand arouses understandable opposition – it is a matter of general observation that people never willingly abandon a libidinal

> position, not even, indeed, when a substitute is already beckoning to them. This opposition can be so intense that a turning away from reality takes place and a clinging to the object through the medium of a hallucinatory wishful psychosis. (Freud, 1917b, pp. 244–245)

He suggests that because of this difficulty, '… its [reality's] orders cannot be obeyed at once. They are carried out bit by bit, at great expense of time and cathectic energy, and in the meantime the existence of the lost object is psychically prolonged' (Freud, 1917b, pp. 244–245).

It is because we are so reluctant to accept the reality of loss that the work of mourning is needed: this is not only painful and arduous but also takes time.

> Each single one of the memories and situations of expectancy which demonstrate the libido's attachment to the lost object is met by the verdict of reality that the object no longer exists; and the ego, confronted as it were with the question whether it shall share this fate, is persuaded by the sum of the narcissistic satisfactions it derives from being alive to sever its attachment to the object that has been abolished. We may perhaps suppose that this work of severance is so slow and gradual that by the time it has been finished the expenditure of energy necessary for it is also dissipated. (Freud, 1917b, p. 255)

Finally, at the conclusion of mourning, the libido that has been withdrawn from the object is freed up so that it can be invested in new relationships. It is precisely this change that is blocked in melancholia and accounts for the chief difference between the two conditions. In other respects, mourning and melancholia are remarkably similar and can be considered to lie on a continuum in which the symptoms become more severe the longer that mourning is delayed.

The Nature of the Melancholic Internal Object

Freud proceeds to a detailed description of the self-reproaches that are characteristic of melancholia.

> The patient represents his ego to us as worthless, incapable of any achievement and morally despicable; he reproaches himself, vilifies himself and expects to be cast out and punished. He abases himself before everyone and commiserates with his own relatives for being connected with anyone so unworthy. … This picture of a delusion of (mainly moral) inferiority is completed by sleeplessness and refusal to take nourishment, and – what is psychologically very remarkable – by an overcoming of the instinct which compels every living thing to cling to life. (Freud, 1917b, p. 246)

From these descriptions, Freud concludes that the denigration of the ego arises from a part of the ego that has been altered by internalisation and identification. Initially he calls this a special agency, which subsequently becomes the super-ego.

> We see how in him one part of the ego sets itself over against the other, judges it critically, and, as it were, takes it as its object. Our suspicion that the critical agency which is here split off from the ego might also show its independence in other circumstances will be confirmed by every further observation. (Freud, 1917b, p. 247)

So, we have one part of the ego, identified with the lost object, looking down and expressing 'dissatisfaction with the ego on moral grounds'. Freud connects this with the normal 'conscience', but observes that it can become diseased and pathological. The pathology can be readily observed in the extreme cruelty with which the self is attacked.

> Following our view of sadism, we should say that the destructive component had entrenched itself in the super-ego and turned against the ego. What is now holding sway in the super-ego is, as it were, a pure culture of the death instinct, and in fact it often enough succeeds in driving the ego into death, if the latter does not fend off its tyrant in time by the change round into mania. (Freud, 1923, p. 53)

The Responses of the Ego to Condemnations from the Super-Ego

Freud describes how in depression the ego submits to the condemnations and concurs with the unfavourable verdict of the super-ego. The patient agrees that he is inferior and accepts his humiliation as appropriate to his lowly status. However, by listening patiently, Freud made yet another striking discovery when he noted that self-reproaches were not only rather loud and persistent but could also be seen to be directed not at the patient but at someone else.

> If one listens patiently to a melancholic's many and various self-accusations, one cannot in the end avoid the impression that often the most violent of them are hardly at all applicable to the patient himself, but that with insignificant modifications they do fit someone else, someone whom the patient loves or has loved or should love. Every time one examines the facts this conjecture is confirmed. So we find the key to the clinical picture: we perceive that the self-reproaches are reproaches against a loved object which have been shifted away from it on to the patient's own ego. (Freud, 1917b, p. 248)

What seems to be happening is that having succumbed to the criticisms of the super-ego, the patient's self-recriminations also express complaints and grievances directed against the injustice of his treatment.

> The behaviour of the patients, too, now becomes much more intelligible. Their complaints are really 'plaints' in the old sense of the word. They are not ashamed and do not hide themselves, since everything derogatory that they say about themselves is at bottom said about someone else. Moreover, they are far from evincing towards those around them the attitude of humility and submissiveness that would alone befit such worthless people. On the contrary, they make the greatest nuisance of themselves, and always seem as though they felt slighted and had been treated with great injustice. All this is possible only because the reactions expressed in their behaviour still proceed from a mental constellation of revolt, which has then, by a certain process, passed over into the crushed state of melancholia. (Freud, 1917b, 248)

It seems to me that Freud is suggesting that two trends are being expressed simultaneously, one in which the self is identified as the inferior worthless object and the other in which the tables are turned, and it is the super-ego that is felt to be at fault and its criticisms viewed as unfair. This complex of attitudes is also found when depression gives way to mania.

Mania

Freud's discussion of mania highlights the importance of triumph and excitement, which serve as a defence against the pain of depression. In depression, the ego is judged as inferior, while in mania the seesaw is triumphantly reversed and it is the object that is subjected to the severity of the judgement. Freud draws attention to the contrast between the high spirits of mania and the low mood and inhibition of depression, but he also asserts that the two conditions are fundamentally similar.

> The impression which several psycho-analytic investigators have already put into words is that the content of mania is no different from that of melancholia, that both disorders are wrestling with the same 'complex', but that probably in melancholia the ego has succumbed to the complex whereas in mania it has mastered it or pushed it aside. (Freud, 1917b, p. 254)

If we remember that Freud found that the self-recriminations in depression were also protests against the unfairness of the criticism, then it may be that triumph is not limited to mania but is also discernible in the depressive phase of the disorder. Freud mentioned that he saw no evidence of triumph in mourning, but Klein (1940) was later to question this conclusion. If we also remember that the apparent self-abasement of the melancholic is also a criticism directed at the super-ego, it may be that the triumph is hidden and indirectly expressed in depression while openly shown in mania. It seems to me that Freud's descriptions point to the idea that a mutual state of grievance between the ego and the super-ego is characteristic of melancholia, whereby each expresses disappointment with the other. In their relationship, sometimes one and sometimes the other is in ascendency, and the reversal from the crushed to the superior state can become a source of excitement and triumph. The mutual grievances and the hostility and triumph associated with them can become so intense that it seems as if a state of chronic warfare develops between the ego and the super-ego in the internal world. When the hostility is enacted in the transference, it can become an important source of impasse in analysis.

Not Being Loved Is Equated with Humiliation and Death

Freud postulates that melancholia, like mourning, is a response to a loss, but the loss is not aways due to the actual loss of an object. To lose the love of the loved object can be as bad as or worse than losing the object itself, and such setbacks occur with those slights and disappointment that are common in all relationships and that may seem catastrophic. 'An object-choice, an attachment of the libido to a particular person, had at one time existed; then, owing to a real slight or disappointment coming from this loved person, the object-relationship was shattered' (Freud, 1917b, pp. 248–249). Slights and disappointments seem relatively mild injuries, but Freud makes clear that to lose the love of a good object can throw the patient into a serious melancholia.

> The fear of death in melancholia only admits of one explanation: that the ego gives itself up because it feels itself hated and persecuted by the super-ego, instead of loved. To the ego, therefore, living means the same as being loved – being loved by the super-ego, which here again appears as the representative of the id. (Freud, 1923, p. 58)

The sense of disappointment suggests an expectation that fails to be met, and the grievances, both those held by the super-ego against the ego and by the ego against the super-ego, are based on comparisons with an ideal of what they ought to be. It is this which gives the super-ego a moral dimension and makes the ego feel condemned and humiliated when it is seen to fail to meet this standard. The idealisation associated with narcissism was a feature of Freud's model of the ego ideal, and it is this idealisation that makes the standard impossible to meet.

Narcissistic Object Relations

Certainly, Freud thought that narcissism was a precondition for the development of melancholia, and in his introduction to 'Mourning and Melancholia', Strachey gave it great weight.

> What enabled Freud to reopen the subject [of melancholia] was, of course, the introduction of the concepts of narcissism and of an ego ideal. The present paper may, indeed, be regarded as an extension of the one on narcissism which Freud had written a year earlier. (Strachey's 'Editor's Note' in Freud, 1917b, p. 240)

It is the narcissistic nature of the relationship in melancholia that makes the withdrawal of libido difficult and binds the self and the object in an identification that interferes with mourning.

> ... the object-choice has been effected on a narcissistic basis, so that the object-cathexis, when obstacles come in its way, can regress to narcissism. The narcissistic identification with the object then becomes a substitute for the erotic cathexis, the result of which is that in spite of the conflict with the loved person the love-relation need not be given up. This substitution of identification for object-love is an important mechanism in the narcissistic affections. (Freud, 1917b, p. 249)

Because the identifications in melancholia are so complex, it may be helpful to make a short diversion and discuss Freud's writings on this topic, which began with his discussion of the Leonardo case (Freud, 1910; Strachey, in Freud 1917b). Here he describes how Leonardo projected his child self into his apprentices, and looked after them as he wished his mother had looked after him.

> The child's love for his mother cannot continue to develop consciously any further; it succumbs to repression. ... he puts himself in her place, identifies himself with her, and takes his own person as a model in whose likeness he chooses the new objects of his love. ... boys whom he loves in the way in which his mother loved him when he was a child. He finds the objects of his love along the path of narcissism, as we say. (Freud, 1910, p. 100)

Later he describes what he calls a narcissistic object-choice.

> They are plainly seeking themselves as a love-object, and are exhibiting a type of object-choice which must be termed 'narcissistic'. In this observation we have the strongest of the reasons which have led us to adopt the hypothesis of narcissism. (Freud, 1914, p. 88)

If we apply these thoughts to the relationship between the self and the internal object, that is between ego and super-ego, then a double identification can be seen to have taken place, something like that described of Leonardo. The ego is split into superior and inferior elements, and in the self-recriminations the ego is identified as the child and the super-ego with the condemning parent. However, as we have seen, in mania, and in a hidden way in depression, the situation is reversed, and the child takes a critical view of the behaviour of the parent.

This kind of whistle-stop survey inevitably fails to do justice to the complexity of Freud's schema for mourning and his hypotheses for the nature of melancholia. It may, however, identify some of the critical findings of which any contemporary model of mourning and melancholia must take account: for example, in mourning, the internalisation and identification as a response to loss; the narcissistic nature of the identification in which libido remains attached to the lost object; the work of mourning required to detach this libido and to allow it to be invested in new objects, and the requirement to apply the verdict of reality to each of the memories associated with the object to confirm that it is irretrievably lost. Freud points out the similarities between mourning and melancholia, and concludes that the chief difference between them is that in melancholia the work of mourning has failed. The self-recriminations show how the internal object is set up above the ego, judging it unfavourably; the ego accepts the unfavourable view but at the same time protests against the unfairness of the judgements. In mania, the protest leads to a reversal of the roles and a triumphant condemnation of the previously revered internalised lost object.

Kleinian and Post-Kleinian Developments

Even though there have been few advances as fundamental as those of Freud, I believe that his findings can be deepened and clarified by the application of more recent formulations. For me the important developments arise from Klein's (1946) descriptions of the splitting and projective identification which affect the constitution of internal objects, and which govern the relationship between them.

Projective Identification Creating a Composite-Object

When Klein introduced the idea of projective identification in 1946, she initiated a new understanding of object relations in which elements of the self and object were interchanged and no longer experienced as separate. Of the numerous accounts of projective identification, I have found those of Sodré (2004), Britton (1998), and Feldman (1992, 1994, 1997) to be most relevant, and these build on the earlier, more pioneering work of Klein (1946, 1952), Rosenfeld (1971, 1983), Bion (1962), Segal (1957), and Joseph (1987). It is important to recognise that projective identification is an umbrella term covering a variety of related mechanisms which alter the perception of both self and object and which interfere with the experience of self and object as separate entities. In one of the common forms of this mechanism, unwanted parts of the self are split off and through projection are felt to have entered the object and have been attributed to it and identified with it. Here it is the object that is identified with the projected fragment which the self has disowned, with the result that the perception of the object is altered and that of the self is depleted. The primary motive for the above type of projective identification is to disown an undesirable quality, that is to evacuate it into the mind of the object, while at other times the mechanism can be motivated by a wish to attack and control the object or even to acquire its properties. Bion (1962) has described how projective identification is not always pathological and can serve as a primitive form of communication in which the mother's capacity to accept and understand the projections plays a crucial role. These different functions commonly operate simultaneously, and their understanding may depend on the analyst's capacity to contain and differentiate the different types. Alongside the projective mechanisms, introjective identifications allow elements of the object to be internalised and incorporated into the ego.

Because of the variety of its applications, the designation *projective identification* is not in itself a sufficient description of this mechanism, and in every individual instance it is necessary to specify what has been projected with what motive and with what consequences.[2] For the purpose of understanding mourning and melancholia, I think it is important to focus on two of the important consequences: first that the perception of both the self and of the object are altered, and second that the object acquires the property of concreteness as the ego's capacity to think symbolically is blocked.

In order to emphasise the effect of projective identification on the nature of the object, it seems appropriate to think of the internal object as a composite-object, with the specific properties that arise from the failure to establish a separateness between self and object.

Concreteness of the Internal Composite-Object

The importance of the composite-object lies partly in the creation of a persecutory super-ego whose severity is increased through the projection of infantile sadism, but partly also because of the important property of concreteness that characterises composite-objects. In depression they commonly appear subjectively as a painful heaviness in which the object is experienced as a mass that exists as a burden in the mind and a pressure in the body. Freud

2 Henri Rey used to say, 'What part of the subject, in what state, situated where in space and time does what, with what motivation, to what part of the object, situated where in space and time, with what consequences for the object and the subject' (personal communication, 1966).

spoke of the shadow of the object falling on the ego, and we might add that along with the darkness cast by the shadow, a heavy burden has been acquired. When the distress is experienced as a somatic rather than a mental pain, it can lead to requests for urgent relief from doctors, which are transferred to the analyst. It is the unbearability of pain of this kind that can drive the patient to suicidal solutions as the only way of getting rid of the problem.

The concrete thinking is also revealed in the demands made by the super-ego of the melancholic for reparation and revenge, which are actual rather than symbolic. Freud showed how the self-reproaches are at the same time reproaches against the object; commonly both self and object feel themselves to have been injured and each demands that the other make good the damage they have done. In this situation it is the concreteness of the demands which makes them so difficult for the patient to bear. This is especially problematic in the demand for reparation and revenge, which at a concrete level are felt to be impossible and can only be satisfied through omnipotence.

It is here that the development of symbolic function can transform the impasse by liberating the use of memory, dreams and phantasy to open up a world of the imagination in which symbolic reparation becomes possible. If the patient is able to think symbolically, contact with the object is retained in the form of memories and symbols and opens up new possibilities that are not always evident to the patient and sometimes not to the analyst. Henri Rey provides an example in a patient who felt that she could do nothing for her mother because she was dead. He suggested that her internal mother could be restored if she became a good mother to her own children and could then imagine her mother's pleasure in her grandchildren.[3] This example shows the need to withdraw libido that has been invested in objects from the past in order to make it available for the future. It illustrates how the object continues to exist in a symbolic form even when its concrete presence has been accepted as lost.

The Withdrawal of Projections as the Work of Mourning

In his emphasis on the withdrawal of libido Freud was using the language of drive theory, which we are now able to supplement with an object relations formulation of the process. The recognition of the lost object as a composite-object means that we can postulate that, in addition to the withdrawal of libido, it is elements of the self that are withdrawn and returned to the ego, thus establishing a separateness between self and object. The verdict of reality can then involve a judgement of what belongs to the self and what belongs to the object, and leads to reassignments in which the self is enriched by regaining the previously disowned elements and the object is viewed more realistically and less distorted by projections.

3 Personal communication, 1966.

Freud had been puzzled as to why the work of mourning should be so extraordinarily painful (1917b, p. 245) and the idea of withdrawing projections provides an image of the painful tearing apart that seems to be required. Henri Rey argued it was necessary to 'render unto the object what belongs to the object, and to the self what belongs to the self'.[4] It is, moreover, understandable that this work must be done piecemeal, and we can imagine that each of the memories and situations of expectancy which demonstrate that both self and object have been altered by projections must be tested by a judgement of reality. With the acceptance that the object is lost, projected elements can be reassigned to the self, while others that had been appropriated can be returned and assigned to the object. The work of mourning requires great effort and suffering, and, most of all, time, but when it is successful the eventual result is a degree of separateness between self and object and a regaining of the capacity to invest in new situations and new object relations.

The Turning Point of Mourning

These changes take place at what we can think of as a turning point in mourning, where the focus of interest which is at first pointed backwards towards the lost object changes direction to look forwards to the future. The investment of libido is reversed, turning a full 180 degrees from the past towards the future and from the previous generation to the next. For this critical change to take place, it is necessary for the object to be accepted as irretrievably lost, and it is this verdict of reality that is so commonly resisted, leaving the mourner trapped with his ghosts, preoccupied with his losses, and unable to move on. This turning point is associated with several interrelated changes. The acceptance of loss, the redirection of libido, and the return of projections are closely related, as is the development of symbolic function.

Obstacles to Mourning

Further contributions of a Kleinian approach help us to clarify various obstacles to mourning and raise the possibility that their understanding can help the melancholic patient to sort out his grievances and move towards accepting his losses. As described in the Introduction, these are the focus of subsequent chapters of the book.

4 Personal communication, 1966.

2 Before and After the Fall

Horizontal and Vertical Object Orientations in the Analysis of a Patient with Grievances[1]

Introduction

In this chapter, the vertical relationship in which the super-ego looks down on the ego is described as an important source of grievance, which blocks mourning. It is traced back to the early trauma of losing an idealised relationship with the mother, experienced as an expulsion from Paradise. The fall establishes a vertical relationship between self and object that comes to be internalised as that between ego and super-ego. Clinical material is presented to show that even though grievances create major obstacles to mourning, they can sometimes soften and allow development to be resumed.

Grievances and Disappointments that Interfere with Mourning

Grievances and disappointments are commonly encountered in analytic work, and are often directed against figures in the patient's family and work environment (Steiner, 1996b; Feldman, 2008; Hoggett, 2018; Anderson, 2024). When revived in the transference, the patient's anger is chiefly directed at the analyst's adoption of what seems to them to be a superior position. They feel disapproved of and looked down upon, and respond in kind, criticising the analyst's attitude and creating a vertical relationship of mutual hostility. Both the patient and the analyst fail to live up to each other's expectations, as both feel aggrieved that their current situation is not the one they deserve, and have a right to expect. Each strives to adopt the moral high ground in a relationship that creates an up-and-down world of either triumph or humiliation. It is such striving for the upper hand that characterises the conflict between the ego and the super-ego in melancholia, where it prevents change by interfering with the work of mourning.

1 The chapter is based on J. Steiner (2025b), Before and After the Fall: Horizontal and Vertical Object Orientations, *The International Journal of Psychoanalysis*, 106: 873–891.

DOI: 10.4324/9781003726135-3

The Trauma of the Loss of the Horizontal Relationship

The distinction I make between the vertical and horizontal is like that made by Juliet Mitchell (2013, 2022), when she differentiated the vertical relationship between parent and child, marked by generational difference, from the horizontal one between siblings who are viewed as similar. The relationship between the parents is also horizontal but at a higher level to that of the children, and it is the gap between the two levels that emphasises differences and can make the infant feel small in relation to the adult. The differences, however, vanish in the universal phantasy of an idealised and timeless love affair with the mother (Steiner, 2018, 2024; Weiss, 2008), in which the infant engages in what is felt to be a horizontal relationship at the parental level. Not only are the differences between the generations ignored, but so too is the fact that the horizontal orientation depends on the willingness of the mother to lift the infant to the breast and hold it there in her arms and later in her gaze. In his narcissistic omnipotence, the infant fails to recognise this dependence, and when the mother looks away or attends to other tasks, it feels dropped and falls to a lowly position exposed to the downward gaze of a vertical scrutiny. The contrast between the vertical and the idealised horizontal relationship can make the fall unbearably humiliating and lead to phantasies of triumphant reversal in which it is the object rather than the self that is looked down upon and despised.

Ignês Sodré[2] put this well in some unpublished comments on an earlier paper, in which I described the idealised relationship as the Garden of Eden Illusion (Steiner, 2018).

> Confrontations over power can often be seen to develop as a result of humiliating disappointments in relation to an idealised object. When the patient has created a phantasy in which he can control an ideal object and identify with it, any response that challenges this may lead to a feeling of catastrophic collapse.
>
> The Ideal Object always causes some humiliation at the moment of the first realisation of separateness because as the object is seen more realistically i.e. no longer as a possession and with the idealisation gone, the Fall is too great from a merging position of 'I'm the breast and the breast is me', to 'I need the breast, which is not me'. This often seems to lead to a realisation that 'it is not uniquely mine either', which is equated with the conviction that 'I am not loved at all.'
>
> Normally the mother's love saves the day, since it creates a link and is felt to rescue the baby from the abyss. But if this fails and the pain, humiliation, and fear are unbearable, the 'horizontal' gap, between self and breast becomes a 'vertical' gap, with only two positions, triumph or

2 It is sad to record the death of Ignês Sodré in 2025. The quotations from her papers and communications testify to her enormous contribution to psychoanalysis.

> humiliation. The longing for love is then replaced by a longing for power. The patient inhabits an up and down universe in which strength fuelled by hatred is idealised and love is seen as weak and contemptible.[3]

Power is sought to deal with the humiliating inferior position in the struggle between the self and the internalised lost object, which becomes that between the ego and the super-ego. As this struggle is played out in the transference, it typically leads to confrontations between patient and analyst.

Of course, there is another current that reflects a loving relationship between the self and the lost object which survives the trauma of the loss and includes feelings of appreciation, loyalty and gratitude. Indeed, it is these feelings that make it so difficult to say goodbye and let the object go. The hostility has not arisen towards a bad object but towards what Ron Britton has called, a 'good object behaving badly',[4] and the hope is that the object will relent, accept that the fault is his and restore the idealisation. The analyst is commonly put in the place of an arbiter of the justice of complaints against someone else, and comes under moral pressure to agree with the patient's view of what happened. The role can be like that of a mother who must arbitrate in a fight between siblings, and if the analyst does not side with the patient, it is the analyst who becomes the focus of the grievance. It is here, then, that the idealised relationship is most under threat, and nothing short of restoring the perfect agreement will satisfy the grievance.

In these circumstances, the fall may even be attributed to treachery and betrayal, and the resentment becomes so intense that it creates the impression of a war between the self and the lost object. Morality becomes more important than reality, as each wants to adopt the super-ego role in which what *should* happen takes priority over what *has* happened. When externalised in the transference, the entrenched grievances lead to confrontations that may create a stuck situation which can dominate an analysis.

Clinical Material

I will use these formulations to look anew at some clinical material from Mr D, a patient previously described, who seemed to be making significant steps towards development after long periods of stasis in a severe depression with obsessional features.[5] He began analysis in his late forties in a terrible crisis. His wife could no longer tolerate his anger-fuelled misery and had asked him to leave, he felt thwarted in his work, and he was suffering from severe pain in his feet that had even led him to seek drastic interventions from surgeons. After a brilliant Oxbridge degree, he had embarked on a series

3 Sodré, personal communication, 2012.

4 Personal communication, 2020.

5 The material has been published previously (Steiner, 2005, 2015, 2020). It has been disguised to protect confidentiality.

of ambitious career moves, each seeming to begin with great success and then coming crashing down in a terrible collapse. They all involved scientific developments directed towards easing deprivation in the Third World, and he had built a significant reputation in his field. He was living alone, with problematic access to his two children, and despite her hostility he was determined to persuade his wife to have him back. He saw his father as a failure professionally and believed, possibly with his mother's connivance, that he was expected to restore the family name and fortune.

At his office, his anger was focussed on a reshuffle in which he had been replaced as director of his project by a colleague I will call Norman, of much inferior scientific ability. This led to a fury with the management that he referred to as 'road rage'.

First Session

Mr D began a Monday session by saying that he was very aware that there were only two weeks left. He was going to say, 'until the break', but that assumed he was coming back, and he might decide to stop. He said he had felt more normal at the weekend, contacting friends and spending time with his parents.

He went on to say that he had also realised things about himself. He had perceived an element of what he could only call snobbism, especially with Norman, and he had realised that he was more comfortable with people of his own class.

He also had to come to terms with his attitude to black people. He had observed that a high proportion of people who drove aggressively were black. He reported that when he gave way to a black driver, they didn't acknowledge him, while he always waved a thank-you when someone gave way to him. He said that he was trying to say this in a way that would prevent me jumping on him and saying that he was racist.

At first, I tried to avoid a confrontation and interpreted his wish to be recognised as someone who opposed racism and snobbism. I noted that he felt he had had a better weekend with friends and family, and I suggested that this may have made him feel more able to face difficult realisations about himself. To this he was impatient and irritable, saying that he simply wanted me to look at the facts. It seemed to take us a long time to get anywhere. Why was I holding back? he asked. I was being too careful and not straightforward.

I thought he was right, and interpreted that he wanted me to face the fact that it was his fury with me that I had been avoiding. I thought that his racism and snobbism arose when he felt that, like Norman, I had an unfair advantage over him.

He disagreed angrily and said he could not see where I got that idea from. It was not prejudice and had nothing to do with the colour of someone's skin or their accent. What made him hostile was how people behaved, for example the fact that Norman took messages and did not acknowledge them. He could not stand the way his views were ignored.

I acknowledged that he had a right to have his views heard, but I also interpreted that the reasonable demand for mutual respect could conceal his wish for our relationship to be symmetrical. He would wave to me if I waved to him. If I accused him of racism, he could feel wronged, and we could not examine the possibility that our relationship did involve differences. I thought that his road rage was a response to those differences that made him feel looked down upon.

Discussion of the First Session

Eventually Mr D's rage became more openly focussed in the transference, and he argued that his protests were not to do with snobbism or racism, as I had been challenged to assert, but were focussed on the way his views were ignored. I eventually realised that, like Norman, I had been taking messages without acknowledging them. Indeed, the protest seemed to have begun when he stated that he might still end his analysis rather than return after the break. This seemed to be an assertion that he was not completely powerless and could resist when he felt controlled by me. I think his rage focussed on his wish for a horizontal relationship of mutuality, where we both gave way to the other's point of view. I think he feared I would remain morally superior, attributing racism to him and denying it in myself.

Second Session

He began a second session with a dream in which he had visited a modern art exhibition. One item was a tree root with small rootlets sticking out and looking untidy. He thought it needed pruning, and he took out some secateurs and cut off a piece of root, which he put in his pocket. He was embarrassed and sidled out of the museum, hoping he would not be seen. Once out of the building he felt relief, thinking, 'They can't do anything to me now.'

He went on to say that the firm's accountants had caught up with him at last over some money he had spent on a project of his own. The firm had paid and were now demanding they be reimbursed. He had obtained a grant for this project but to get the grant he had to write a report, which he kept putting off. The memo asking 'Where is the money?' had made him panic. He feared the need to write the report would blight his summer, and he was tempted to pay the money out of his own pocket. He knew they would find out, and he asked himself, what is the worst they can do? He hadn't stolen the money; it was all accounted for.

Returning to his dream, he said there was someone with him in the museum. He thought perhaps it was Norman, and the dream ended back in the office,where Norman leaned forwards and brazenly picked up Mr D's coffee and drank it. In his dream, he had exploded in a rage of resentment.

I interpreted that, as in the earlier session, he was acknowledging that he could be provocative, and that in his dream he seemed to be snipping at my work. He said he was reminded of some secateurs which he had come across in his flat yesterday. He always deadheads the flowers on his patio.

I interpreted that, as with Norman and his coffee, he felt that I helped myself to his ideas and developed them in my way without including him. However, I added that once he had clipped the root in his dream, he seemed to have become aware that it was not his and he had become embarrassed and anxious that he would be found out.

He agreed and went back to the dispute with Norman. He had complained that Norman was trying to cut him out of decision-making. He was going to demand to know if the office was hierarchical or collaborative. Norman had sent a memo as if it had come jointly from them both. Mr D had replied, 'No, this is not collaboration, it is you exercising authority.'

I interpreted that he hated the hierarchical relationship between us that made him feel looked down upon, and that his hatred had led him to vandalise the exhibit in the museum and made him feel ashamed and afraid of being caught.

He became angry again and attacked my use of the word vandalise, which he said was quite wrong. People who spoiled GM crops were not getting pleasure from destroying but trying to get their protest heard. I was able to link this with his feeling of being wrongly accused of stealing the grant money, and that he did not think his attack on the root in the museum was wrong. 'Everything was accounted' for implied that he was entitled to take the rootlet. Perhaps he felt it was *his* analysis that I was showing off in the museum, with his contribution ignored. I suggested that the report which he found so difficult to write was an account of our work, perhaps including who had contributed what, and that it meant distinguishing what belonged to him and what belonged to me. It was this struggle that was so painful and would plague him in the break.

After a silence he began thinking of the time he had failed his test for a motorbike licence in Germany. He was outraged because the bit he had failed involved moving slowly between cones with a pillion rider. What was unfair was that this was a skill he would never need to use, and he had been riding a bike competently for years. It was those bloody Germans! They thought they owned the roads! Then after a pause he said, 'I suppose you could say that the Germans do own their own roads.'

Discussion of the Second Session

The contentious issue in this session centred on his snipping off the rootlet from the exhibit in the gallery. First, he linked it with deadheading flowers, which implied that the pruning was beneficial. Later he connected it with Norman brazenly taking his coffee, and I thought he felt that I show off my work and help myself to his ideas without acknowledging him. Like his accountants, I was led to think there might be some stealing going on, and I even described the snipping of the root as vandalism. I thought this was an enactment on my part when I felt he failed to take responsibility for attacking the rootlet and it brought his rage into the transference in his claim that, like attacks on GM crops, he was making a protest. His argument supported his view that he had done nothing wrong, but he did admit that to put things straight he would have to write a report, and it was here that the blockage lay. The report was so difficult because it forced him to sort out what belonged to him and what belonged to me, and I think he demanded that I do the same and acknowledge his contribution. His rage was again with the hierarchical relationship, in which he felt he was placed at a lower level and that his protest was misunderstood as an attack.

I think his rage with the motorbike test was connected to his anger at the way I set the rules of the analysis, like the session times, the fees, and the use of the couch. There was probably also a reference to me sitting behind him like a pillion rider and a relief that he could discard this arrangement when the analysis was over. In the meantime, he did not feel he was an equal partner, and all he could do was protest at the injustice. When he accepted that the Germans did own their own roads, he seemed to admit that I was entitled to determine the analytic setting as long as he was entitled to protest against it. This seemed to be a softening of his grievances against me, and I think represented a turning point in his attitude.

The material illustrated how our confrontations were part of the up-and-down world in which a vertical relationship prevailed, and he felt either unjustly judged and humiliated, or triumphantly able to turn the tables and insist I was the one in the wrong.

Third Session

Some time later, as we were nearing the end of his long and often contentious analysis, Mr D decided to accept an invitation to give a talk at a business convention in Germany, which meant that he would have to miss his Friday session.

He began in a distraught state explaining that a catastrophe had happened. His wife had suggested that he should help his son find a job and had implied that he could pull strings through his contacts in high places. When he did so, at the cost of considerable effort and embarrassment, it had led to disaster. Instead of winning approval from his son, he had been accused of interfering and of trampling on his independence. It indicated that there was something wrong with his thinking, that wires were connected up wrongly in his head, and that he was beyond being saved. Perhaps, he added, this was revenge for a feeling of complacency in recent weeks, when he had thought he had pleased his wife through his work in their garden. Things had been going deceptively well and he had felt good, but had then pulled the rug out from under himself, and everything had come crashing down.

The depressive self-reproaches were loud but shorter lasting than usual. Later in the session he recovered somewhat and asked himself why he had collapsed so readily in the face of his wife's demands and then of his son's accusations. He wished he had been able to stand up for his belief that pulling strings was not the way to help his son but he also felt that he had not done anything so terrible. I thought he could see that his internal strength had collapsed, and he wanted my support to stand up against a demanding and unjust internal voice functioning as a severe critic, with which he had felt obliged to comply.

I also linked the patient's description of disaster with his anxiety over the business trip he was to take to Germany the next day, and I interpreted that he was trying to see if I would adopt a critical stance and imply that he should not miss a session for his trip. He could then claim that I thought that missing a session would be a disaster. When I seemed to respect his decision, he felt more able to make judgements and stand up for himself.

Fourth Session

After the weekend in Germany, Mr D came back in a different mood. He said that he had received a long apologetic e-mail from his son and that he had watched a television documentary about the D-day landings in Normandy. His father had taken part in the invasion, and Mr D realised how traumatic it must have been. He thought this was probably why his father had never taken him camping and maybe why his father had an antipathy to all things German. When Mr D gave his talk in Germany the previous Friday, he had felt excited when the Germans were impressed by his work, and he wondered if this had something to do with his rivalry with his father.

I suggested that he might think that, like his father, I – and psychoanalysis – had a history connected with Germany in the war, and that, like his father, I might be hurt if he embraced Germany with too much enthusiasm. He said that he had been thinking of psychoanalysis as German, and then had realised it was Austrian and Jewish. He then remembered a remarkable day when he had been sitting in a café in Germany, near the French border. He had had a good meal and some wine, and had written some notes which he thought of as his personal manifesto. This piece of writing was long and involved, but it had flowed easily. If he were to look at it now he might see it as nonsense. He added that he felt controlled by his father, and this made him angry. But when he was watching the documentary, he was moved when they said that there would soon be no veterans left to attend the celebrations.

I interpreted that he was now more aware of the end of the analysis, which linked to a time when I would no longer be here. This created a conflict. He could easily see me as controlling and as demanding that he submit to my authority. Then, if he rebelled, he feared that it would take the form of a terrible triumph connected with Germany and the war.

He agreed that his longing for rebellion was a manic sort of freedom and was dangerous. He knew it was connected with fascism and power. He added that as his father was getting older, he himself was finding it easier to accept that when one generation passes money on to the next, they will not be there to see how it is spent.

I suggested that he had been afraid that taking the long weekend for the business trip could have led him to experience feelings of power, superiority, and triumph in identification with fascist ideology. However, as he had recovered from his collapse, he was less convinced that his actions and phantasies were a disaster and did not believe they would lead to a catastrophic loss of my support. Now, he seemed more aware that after the analysis ended, I would not be there to supervise how he used what he had gained from it. Mr D said that he had noticed a change at a recent family occasion when his father put his arm over his mother's shoulder. Previously he was sure he saw her cringe when this happened, but this time he noticed she leant towards him.

I interpreted that he now felt safer with me, and that I and my relationship with psychoanalysis had survived his long weekend in Germany, despite his excited feelings of triumph when his omnipotence was stimulated. He said that he had a number of promising projects in the pipeline, but he found it difficult to judge if they were real or just excited and mad. I interpreted that what had changed was that now he would try to judge these for himself rather than provoke me to criticise them.

Discussion of Third and Fourth Sessions

It seems to me that the catastrophe that followed the collapse of his plan to help with his son's job led to typically melancholic self-reproaches in which he accepted all of the blame. The collapse followed a manic triumph connected with his talk in Germany, but on this occasion it was short-lived, and he recovered a capacity to stand up for himself and for what he believed was right. Thinking of his manifesto, he remembered that psychoanalysis was Austrian and Jewish, and this made him realise that I might feel distressed and even threatened if he espoused Nazi ideology. These thoughts released feelings of sorrow, which connected with his realisation that the analysis was going to end soon. Now he might review his judgements and perhaps see his manifesto as nonsense, and he could bring a picture of his parents together in a better relationship.

I thought we could understand that he could not resist turning to phantasies of triumph and revenge, which reversed the feelings of humiliation he had experienced when he felt very small and needy, and when he collapsed. Then, any phantasy that made him feel superior provided relief and excitement. This meant that he accepted that there were times when he identified with a Nazi superiority that normally he would vigorously oppose, just as he did those of snobbism and racism. This admission represented taking back into himself elements that he normally projected into others and had become more possible as he saw me as someone who might similarly acknowledge traits I was ashamed of in myself. It seemed to me that his anger, while still easily revived, became moderated by feelings of sorrow and regret.

General Discussion

The opening stanza of Milton's *Paradise Lost* exemplifies the widely held beliefs that make mourning the loss of the ideal so difficult.

> Of Mans First Disobedience, and the Fruit
> Of that Forbidden Tree, whose mortal taste
> Brought Death into the World, and all our woe,
> With loss of Eden, till one greater Man
> Restore us, and regain the blissful Seat,
> Sing Heav'nly Muse [...]
>
> (1.6)

Not only is the expulsion from Eden seen as a disaster, but the promise of a return to Paradise is kept alive by the poet. Reviewing this account of the expulsion from Eden, Hanna Segal (2007) proposed that the loss which Milton sees as the source of 'all our woes' involved nothing more than the acceptance of reality in place of the illusion of a timeless paradise. The situation is expressed in what Akhtar (1996) has called 'if-only' and 'someday' phantasies, commonly observed in both patients and analysts. The 'if-only' version suggests that we could still be in Paradise if only the loss had been avoided, while 'someday' looks forward to a time when Paradise is regained. The universal appeal of utopian societies, whether religious or political, attests to our reluctance to face the facts of life (Money-Kyrle, 1968, 1971) of which the reality of ageing and death are perhaps the most difficult. Yet it is this loss of the idea of perfection that must be accepted and mourned if we are to live in the real world and suffer the pains and pleasures of reality.

Is it Possible for the Melancholic to Mourn?

If it is a failure to mourn that characterises the melancholic, it is natural to ask what might enable the patient to recover and address the work of mourning with greater success. What could enable the patient to relinquish grievances, accept the reality of loss, and begin the task of separating self from object? Freud was aware that even in normal mourning the task can be painful and difficult, and it seems doubly so when the grievances that establish melancholia have become entrenched.

Yet change does sometimes occur, even though we do not often understand how or why. Nor do our contemporary models offer theoretical or practical advice on how to foster mourning. It is a sobering thought that more than a hundred years have passed since the publication of 'Mourning and Melancholia', and Freud's classic findings have not been significantly bettered. What *has* emerged, with the help of contemporary object relations models, is a better understanding of mental mechanisms which explain some of the obstacles to mourning, obstacles which lead to the stuck situations so typical of melancholia. For me, in particular, it is Klein's formulation of splitting and projective identification (1946) that allows the complexity of the relationship between the self and the lost object to be detailed, and clarifies the mechanisms behind the work of mourning (Joseph, 1987; Feldman, 1992; Ogden, 1979; Rosenfeld, 1971; Sandler, 1987; Sodré, 2004).

Projective Identification Governing Narcissistic Relationships with the Super-Ego

Freud (1917b) recognised that relationships in melancholia were narcissistic, involving love, not for a separate object, but for a self that has been projected into the object. These relationships can be better understood if we make a distinction between normal and pathological projective identification, thinking that normally projective identification is used flexibly and reversibly. It serves as a model for empathy, when we transiently put ourselves into another's shoes; as a primitive means of communication (Bion, 1962; Joseph 1987); and helps us get rid of difficult experiences at times of stress. In the pathological form that characterises melancholia, the parts of the self that are split off and projected into objects become welded together into pathological organisations that become difficult or impossible to reverse (Rosenfeld, 1971; Steiner, 1993b). This means that the internalised lost object that comes to function as a severe super-ego is a composite-object, which has been altered by projections. In such composite-objects, perceptions of the object are distorted through the projections they contain, and the self is also distorted by introjected elements from the object.

In addition to the misrepresentations, this mixing up of self and object has another important consequence, namely that concrete thinking comes to characterise the relationship. Symbolic function, which depends on the ability to tolerate separateness and absence, has failed to develop or has reverted to the concrete, and the object retains a presence in the mind, as if it were the actual object rather than its representation (Segal, 1957). The lost object thus comes to reside internally as a solid presence, burdening the mind, and often experienced as a pain or heaviness in the body. The patient makes concrete demands that the analysis free him of this unfair burden, and he feels that the demands made on him by the super-ego, especially those calling for reparation and revenge, are equally concrete and unreasonable.

The Work of Mourning as the Withdrawal of Libido

Freud indicated that the work of mourning, first and foremost, requires the patient to register and accept the reality of the loss so that a separateness between self and object can be established. He formulated this in terms of a withdrawal of libido which had become fixed to the lost object and had to be detached from it.

'Reality-testing has shown that the loved object no longer exists, and it proceeds to demand that all libido shall be withdrawn from its attachments to that object. This demand arouses understandable opposition' (Freud, 1917b, p. 244).

Freud was puzzled as to why the process should be so extraordinarily painful.

> Each single one of the memories and expectations in which the libido is bound to the object is brought up and hyper-cathected, and detachment of the libido is accomplished in respect of it. Why this compromise by which the command of reality is carried out piecemeal should be so extraordinarily painful is not at all easy to explain in terms of economics. It is remarkable that this painful unpleasure is taken as a matter of course by us. The fact is, however, that when the work of mourning is completed the ego becomes free and uninhibited again. (Freud, 1917b, p. 245)

The Work of Mourning as the Withdrawal of Projections

In his emphasis on the withdrawal of libido Freud was using the language of drive theory, which we are now able to supplement with an object relations formulation of the process. The recognition that the lost object is a composite-object with elements of the self projected into it means that we can postulate that, in addition to the withdrawal of libido, the work of mourning enables these elements to be withdrawn and returned to the self (Steiner, 1993b). Freud's observations remain pertinent, and we can adapt Freud's words to suggest that 'each single one of the memories and expectations in which *parts of the self* are bound to the object is brought up and hyper-cathected, and detachment of the self is accomplished in respect of it.'

We can also accept that the command of reality is carried out piecemeal, and suggest that part of the reason the process is so extraordinarily painful is because, when it is viewed concretely, the separation is felt as an agonising tearing apart of flesh from flesh. We can also agree with Freud that the work of mourning frees up the ego, but can add that the reassignments mean that the self is enriched by gaining the previously disowned elements, and the object is viewed more realistically and less distorted by projections. Equally important is the fact that it is also this withdrawal of projections that confers the enormous advantages of symbolic function, which can allow access to the world of the imagination and enable symbolic reparation to replace concrete repair.

The Obstacles to Mourning

While entrenched grievance can lead to stuck states (Anderson, 2024), change does sometimes occur, and in the sessions I have described above, the patient's grievances did seem to soften to allow a degree of mourning to take place. However, what led to the change was not clear, and it is a striking fact that this often remains the case despite Freud's monumental work and all the progress that has been achieved since. Much remains to be understood, and it may be possible to do little more than point to some of the factors that facilitate or block the relinquishment of grievance and liberate the capacity to mourn.

The Vertical Orientation and the Up-and-Down World

I have tried to show that the task of mourning becomes substantially more difficult when grievance becomes entrenched and creates a vertical relationship in an up-and-down world of humiliation and triumph. I have also argued that the vertical can be better understood if it is traced back to the collapse of the illusion of an idealised horizontal relationship. Such descriptions can remind us of the allure of the horizontal, and the painful trauma of its loss, which may enable the analyst better to identify and empathise with the patient's plight and to recognise the pull towards superiority in the vertical relationship.

In the communication from Sodré quoted above, she suggests that 'Normally the mother's love saves the day, since it creates a link and is felt to rescue the baby from the abyss.'[6] But for the infant to be rescued from his lowly position after the fall, the mother must stoop down to floor level so that, at least temporarily, baby and mother can enjoy a horizontal relationship. It seems right for the analyst to try to approach the patient in his lowly position after the fall and accept the common ground between them. The patient may then be able to accept the invitation to rejoin the family, and both patient and analyst can gradually establish their rightful place in its hierarchy. Such a move often serves as a reassurance that the patient can be loved, but as Feldman points out (1993), it lacks conviction unless the reality of the situation is preserved. The patient may still find it difficult to believe that the analyst's care, like the mother's love, can extend to others without diminishing himself, and moreover, that the differences between them have not been abolished. The analyst's wish to preserve privacy and withhold information about personal issues is a major provocation to the patient's wish for symmetry. If the provocative elements of difference are understood and common elements are not ignored, the hardness of hatred can sometimes soften and release feelings of sorrow and regret. The suffering and terrible wastage of grievance may then be recognised, and moves towards mourning become possible.

Erotisation of Grievance

Many of the other factors that interfere with mourning are connected with the vertical relationship and were, to varying degrees, observable in the case of Mr D. An example is the way a grievance and the vertical orientation may be held onto because of a particular kind of pleasure associated with triumph. The shift of the seesaw from an inferior to a superior position in which

6 Personal communication, 2012.

humiliation is inflicted rather than suffered seems to have a special quality that readily becomes erotised and can exert an addictive hold, which makes the grievance difficult to give up. Stoller (1975) has described how the erotisation may take an explicit form as a pornographic scenario involving humiliation, and Feldman (2008) has described how the patient may come to nurse their grievance and get gratification from feeling wronged.

Grievances commonly lead to withdrawal into a silent resentment in which the subject gets pleasure from the role of victim and the phantasies of revenge remain private. A more open expression of rage can be very frightening but at least allows the resentment to come out in the open and the damage to be more clearly observed. The secret grievance may in fact be even more destructive when it is not fully expressed. This seemed to be the case when Mr D was able to speak about his road rage and focus his hostility in the transference where it could be analysed.

Meanness, Generosity, and the Anal World

It is not always apparent that to release an object and allow it to die can be an act of generosity. In the vertical relationship, the self and the object each restrict the freedom of the other through their demands to be kept alive, remembered, and obeyed. Allowing the object to be free includes the freedom to have an independent mind and to make independent choices, which may involve other members of the family and other priorities. When such freedom is too threatening, the patient may turn to exercising a possessive control, which is associated with anal phantasies. Holding on to the lost object internally may appear as a type of meanness in which the object is cruelly imprisoned and alternatively squeezed and released. Freud made the symbolic equation of faeces = gift = money, and described the anal triad of orderliness, parsimony, and obstinacy (Freud, 1908), in which sadistic control may be associated with phantasies of the object imprisoned inside the anal canal. The object may then be identified with faeces, and giving and withholding linked to what Abraham thought of as anal-retentive and -expulsive phases (Abraham, 1924). Again, these sado-masochistic phantasies are commonly erotised and make it more difficult to relinquish control and liberate the object.

As self-confidence grows, more resources are felt to exist, and an increasing capacity for generosity makes it possible to allow the object more freedom. It is then no longer so vital to possess and control the object and the grievances can afford to soften, as if the sphincters relax and the object is released. Indeed, withdrawing projections can be thought of as an act of generosity, since it liberates objects to be themselves.

The longing to soften is expressed by Hamlet in his first great soliloquy when he proclaims:

> O that this too too solid flesh would melt,
> Thaw, and resolve itself into a dew!
> (*Hamlet* 1.2.129–130)

But softness is viewed as feminine and shameful, and Hamlet fears it will weaken his promise to his father to pursue revenge.

> Then what I have to do
> Will want true colour, tears perchance for blood.
> (*Hamlet* 3.4.132–133)

To exchange the blood of revenge for the tears of sorrow is seen as a betrayal of chivalric values; it is obedience to his father that makes it difficult to accept his loss. At this point Hamlet cannot be disloyal, but later, as he detaches himself from his father, he is able to make a generous gesture and liberate them both as he accepts his own death (Steiner, 2023c).

Generosity and Gratitude

Perhaps the most important barrier to generosity is envy, since it is especially the image of the bountiful mother's freedom to dispense her love as she wishes that so frustrates infantile omnipotence. I have always thought that Klein should have juxtaposed envy and generosity rather than envy and gratitude (Klein, 1957, 1975). Of course, gratitude is an important expression of love but, in contrast to generosity, it reinforces the link to the lost object and encourages a sense of loyalty which may make relinquishment more difficult. For the analyst, the deepest form of gratitude is not the expression of thanks but to see their patients successfully separate and get on with their lives. Gratitude involves good feelings towards good elements in the object, but it is possible to be generous with a variety of emotions and liberate hatred as well as love. As the need for control is lessened, freedom of thought is enhanced, including a willingness to disagree and rebel. Both gratitude and generosity are especially important at times of parting, and to observe a shift away from grievance and meanness towards generosity is one of the most gratifying elements of a successful analysis. Mr D seemed to make a shift in this direction when he acknowledged that the Germans do own their own roads, in which I thought he was generously allowing me to own my own consulting room and to do analysis in my own way.

Attachment and Detachment Throughout Development

Analysts have tended to emphasise the making of connections and given less attention to the need to break them. They often use the baby's relationship with the breast as a model of the transference, and this has perhaps led them to concentrate more on attachment to the object and less on the need for detachment from it. We have, for example, become concerned with patients who are difficult to reach (Joseph, 1975) rather than the equally important problem of patients who are difficult to part from.

Mourning has chiefly been studied in relation to death and bereavement and has not always been considered to play an important role early in life.

Losses, however, are common in any relationship, and every developmental advance involves letting go of the old and embracing the new. The old and familiar has to be relinquished and mourned so that libido can be invested into new relationships and, to develop fully, the inevitable resistance to change has to be overcome. This process can be seen if we follow the various stages of separation-individuation described by Mahler (1972), in which the pain of loss occurs in separations such as those of weaning, sleeping in a separate room, going to school, leaving home, and eventually facing the loss of loved ones through their inevitable death. Each of the changes may be resented and treated as a trauma, and each may revive early wounds and accentuate grievance that may set up a vertical relationship.

The Container as Exoskeleton

Bion (1962) introduced the important idea of containment with his suggestion that the infant projects its anxieties into the mother, where they are relieved through her understanding. Bion seems to be describing an ideal situation which depends on the availability of a receptive space in the mother's mind, and he puts this down to her capacity for reverie. This loose quality of her attention means that her thoughts can be interrupted by communication from the infant and she can be available to respond to projections and understand them. When the capacity for reverie is missing, projections may be blocked and anxiety may be unrelieved, perhaps even made worse. The important maternal quality required seems to be a loose kind of thinking that is not too preoccupied with any particular need. If the mother's mind is filled with some definite project, even, Bion suggests, when this project is the wish to help the infant, her reverie is not free, and she is unable to receive projections. Sometimes the mother relieves anxiety through the provision of an external shell or carapace, producing what can be thought of as a fortress mentality. Bad things are projected outside the walls, and the hard shell protects the soft infant. In these situations, safety is provided at the expense of freedom, and the containing object is introjected as a complex composite-object which relieves anxiety but is difficult to let go of.

It is not uncommon to find patients who feel trapped inside the containing object, which they experience as possessive and controlling, like Henri Rey's patients referring to the psychiatric hospital as a brick mother providing safety without feeling.[7]

7 Henri Rey, personal communication, 1966.

The Internalising of Paternal Support in the Form of a Backbone

Rey likened the immature infant to a soft-bodied invertebrate like a mollusc, which needs the rigid containment of a shell to survive.[8] As development proceeds, however, the infant finds the exoskeleton restrictive and needs to emerge from the shell to enjoy freedom of movement. In order to face the anxieties of the outside world an internal source of strength is required, which Rey thought of as the mental equivalent of a backbone or spinal column, the development of which was such a significant evolutionary advance. With the help of paternal support, the infant is able to leave the maternal container but may need to return if anxiety becomes too great. The infant may feel trapped inside the object and panicky outside it, creating what Rey called the claustro-agoraphobic dilemma (Rey, 1994; Finkelstein and Weiss, 2022).

How the hardness of the external shell becomes internalised as the bony skeleton is far from understood, but the shell may be felt to soften and become a pliable skin, while the strength is somehow incorporated internally as a backbone. Both maternal and paternal sources of strength are needed, and it may be the relationship between them and their ability to support each other that is a critical factor.

The image of Mr D's father putting his arm around his mother seemed to restore his father as a more potent figure that became internalised, and helped Mr D to become the stronger father which he longed to be. Once again mourning seems to be involved, because internal strength is required to face the anxiety of letting go.

The Limitation of What Can Be Achieved in Analysis

Because of the relative weakness of the infant, the triumphant phantasies that give him the upper hand in the vertical relationship are commonly based on omnipotence, and sometimes on alliances with omnipotent objects such as Rosenfeld's narcissistic gangs (1971). Omnipotence may be necessary to avoid being crushed and to find the confidence to rebel and escape from a tyrannical super-ego, but ultimately it must be relinquished and mourned if grievance is to be transformed into sorrow and mourning allowed to proceed.

Segal has argued that it is not only necessary to relinquish the object for mourning to proceed, but that the omnipotence with which the object is controlled and possessed must also be relinquished and mourned.[9] Moreover, she adds that before it can be given up, we must admit we have been omnipotent and acknowledge the enormous pleasure that omnipotence provides. Eventually, the advantages of living in conformity with the facts of life in

8 Henri Rey, personal communication, 1966.
9 Personal communication, 1997.

the real world may outweigh the pleasures of omnipotence, but the choice is never easy and is commonly incomplete. Giving up omnipotence means accepting limitations and finding a rightful place in the family hierarchy in place of the superior and inferior positions of the vertical relationship. Such a change is more readily accepted if symbolic function can allow the world of imagination and phantasy to be distinguished from that of concrete action. Then, dreams of idyllic romance or of triumphant revenge can continue to be enjoyed after their concrete realisations have been abandoned and mourned.

The analyst also has to accept his personal limitations as well as those of psychoanalysis in general. He must endure the feelings of helplessness when progress in the analysis seems to stall, and he has to accept his own excursions into omnipotence especially in his therapeutic zeal towards his patients.

A Note on the Value of Hatred When Grievance Is Justified

Finally, it seems worth remembering that while development requires the eventual acceptance and mourning of loss, there are times when such acceptance is premature. It is not always right to accept loss and mourn it if there is still a chance that the loss may be averted. It is important to be able to protest and fight against injustice and exploitation, and hatred and hostility may clearly serve important functions (Harari, 2022).

In times of war, it is said that truth is the first casualty, but the ability to think symbolically is also vulnerable and equally likely to become a casualty. Concrete thinking enables blame to be projected into the enemy, which helps to justify the aggression that may be necessary for survival. When we are attacked it may be important to fight back, but this means that thinking becomes concrete and truth is of necessity distorted. Responsibility and guilt may have to be set to one side until peace enables symbolic thinking to be ventured once more. A similar concreteness plays an important role in the battles that arise between the ego and the super-ego, and may be needed at those times when threats and persecutions mean that softness and sorrow are too dangerous to contemplate. There is always a time for accepting loss, but not when there is unfinished business that is still to be concluded.

Chivalric values such as courage, loyalty, and gratitude play an important role when external dangers threaten; they link us to our forebears and help us to obey the concrete sacrifices demanded in times of war. When an opportunity for peace arises, and this is true in analysis as it is in war, we must weigh up the costs. This was finely expressed by John Alderdice, in relation to the Good Friday Agreement that brought peace to Northern Ireland, when he said: 'If we find a way to peace we will feel we have betrayed our fathers and grandfathers – if we don't, we will have betrayed our children.'[10]

10 Personal communication, 7 February 2025.

3 Mourning in Hamlet

Turning Ghosts into Ancestors[1]

Introduction

Extracts from Shakespeare's *Hamlet* are used to show how obstacles to mourning may arise from the persistent demands of melancholic internal objects like a ghost demanding repair and revenge. It is only with the development of symbolic function as a result of separateness between self and object that reparation becomes possible and ghosts are turned into ancestors.

I begin these thoughts about mourning with a quote by the singer Bruce Springsteen from a podcast he shared with Barack Obama.

> The trick is you have to turn your ghosts into ancestors. Ghosts haunt you. Ancestors walk alongside you and provide you with comfort and a vision of life that's going to be your own. My father walks alongside me as my ancestor now. It took a long time for that to happen. (Springsteen and Obama, 2021, 33:52)

The phrase, 'Turning ghosts into ancestors' is derived from the work of the American psychoanalyst Hans Loewald (1960) and is used to describe a major achievement in analysis that can allow arrested development to be resumed. I think Loewald believed that progress became blocked through the presence of concrete internal objects that haunt the patient with their demands, and that the patient can be freed up to resume development if the ghosts can be transformed into their symbolic counterparts and take their place in the past as ancestors.

The process by which this is achieved involves mourning that is taken to its conclusion, in which the object is accepted as irretrievably dead and buried.

Eventually we have to be parted from our ghosts, but first they must be brought alive.

1 Based on J. Steiner (2023c), Mourning in Hamlet: Turning Ancestral Ghosts into Ancestors, *The International Journal of Psychoanalysis*, 104: 1025–1041.

DOI: 10.4324/9781003726135-4

Summoning the Ghosts from the Deep

I think of ghosts as primitive persecuting figures that are buried deep in the unconscious and that emerge in times of crisis, as if summoned by contemporary bloodshed. Both Freud and Klein saw such figures as permanent fixtures, separate from the normal super-ego and not alterable through experience. We can only be freed of our preoccupation with them if they can be buried once more and overlaid by less primitive mental developments. Freud saw them as immortal, like the 'legendary Titans'.

> These wishes in our unconscious, ever on the alert and, so to say, immortal, remind one of the legendary Titans, weighed down since primaeval ages by the massive bulk of the mountains which were once hurled upon them by the victorious gods and which are still shaken from time to time by the convulsion of their limbs. (Freud, 1900b, p. 553)

Klein had a similar view:

> These extremely dangerous objects give rise, in early infancy, to conflict and anxiety within the ego; but under the stress of acute anxiety they, and other terrifying figures, are split off in a manner different from that by which the superego is formed and are relegated to the deeper layers of the unconscious. (Klein, 1958, pp. 86–87)

Freud's primitive wishes and Klein's dangerous objects both suggest that the persecutory contents of the unconscious, which I connect with ghosts, cannot be got rid of. They can only be buried and perhaps overlaid by their symbolic counterparts. The relationship with the lost object has to be worked through, but before this can happen a connection with current conflicts must be made. In Freud's words, the ghosts are summoned from the deep by the 'smell of blood'.

> If I may use a simile, they are only capable of annihilation in the same sense as the ghosts in the underworld of the Odyssey – ghosts which awoke to new life as soon as they tasted blood. (Freud, 1900b, footnote p. 553)

Freud is referring to the scene in which Odysseus summoned the ghosts of the dead by sacrificing two sheep. The ghosts were greedy for blood, and only after they had drunk were they able to speak to him. Quite what Freud meant by the taste of blood is not obvious, but it seems to me possible that ghosts arise from the unconscious when they smell the blood of a contemporary grievance. When this matches the patient's own grievance, the ghosts resurface to haunt the ego with their demands. When they come alive, they behave just like the concrete objects of melancholia, full of reproaches and concrete demands. The patient wishes he could be free of them but finds that they cannot be got rid of.

In part, this failure is due to the concrete thinking of the melancholic, which creates a major obstacle to the completion of mourning. While the factors that enable symbolism to develop are as yet only partially understood, it is clear that they have something to do with the work of mourning, which requires the object to be recognised as dead so that libido can be withdrawn from it. Freud recognised the importance of this move, but was also aware that such withdrawal of libido could be extremely painful and that it demanded a 'great expense of time and cathectic energy' (Freud, 1917b, p. 245).

We can understand this disinvestment better if we think of it as involving a reversal of projective identification (Steiner, 1996a), which is also discussed in Chapters 1 and 2 of this book. In the course of mourning, it is not just libido but parts of the self that are returned to the ego. Elements of the self that were previously lost through projective identification are returned, and in the process self and object become more separate. Sometimes the disinvestment seems to leave wounds behind, as if the object is torn away from the self, and the pain, moreover, needs to be repeated as each of the memories of the lost object are subjected to the verdict of reality. However, when this dis-identification *is* allowed to happen, a new and enormously important capacity to symbolise becomes available (Segal, 1957), which allows us to participate in the world of the imagination. We are then able to make use of dreams and fantasies and, in particular, to make symbolic reparation rather than concrete repair.

The Turning Point of Mourning

These changes take place at what we can think of as a turning point in mourning, where the focus of interest which is at first pointed backwards towards the lost object changes direction to look forward to the future. The investment of libido is reversed, turning a full 180 degrees from the past towards the future and from the previous generation to the next. For this critical change to take place, it is necessary for the object to be accepted as irretrievably dead; it is this verdict of reality that is so commonly resisted, leaving the mourner trapped with his ghosts, preoccupied with his losses, and unable to move on.

The Interruption of Mourning by Grievance

This paper arises from a reading of Hamlet in which I was struck that the conflicts faced by Hamlet are similar to those of a bereaved person in the course of mourning. I hope it is clear that this paper is not a literary study but rather tries to use Shakespeare to help us to understand mourning. Oscar Wilde (1854–1900) is often credited with wondering if Hamlet critics were 'really mad, or only pretending to be', although the quotation may be apocryphal, and I have tried to resist pretending to be a learned critic.

In this wonderful play we can follow both the identification that Hamlet makes with his father and his struggle to shed the identification to discover his own identity. Shakespeare offers us a unique insight into the mind of his most intelligent and inward-looking character, which allows us to understand better how the lost object is first identified with and internalised, and then how this identification can be reversed, with the loss accepted and worked through.

Shakespeare shows us how the failure to mourn leaves his hero at the mercy of ghosts who persecute him with their demands, (Shapiro, 2005; Bloom 1999), much like those of the concrete objects characteristic of melancholia.

Hamlet returns home to Denmark to attend his father's funeral, and we see both his attempts to face his loss and his repeated departures from this goal, which are chiefly driven by grievance against his mother and stepfather. Then, when the ghost of his father appears on the ramparts with demands for revenge, he is unable to resist, since they coincide so precisely with his own wishes. The father's hatred is directed towards his brother Claudius who has taken his life and his queen. This hatred coincides with the very same desire for revenge in Hamlet, who has lost his place as his mother's favourite and his father's successor. It seems that identification with a parent is particularly difficult to resist when parental grievances coincide with personal grievances.

How Long Should We Mourn?

At the beginning of the play Hamlet's mother criticises him for remaining too long in his grief, while he responds with outrage at her failure to give grief sufficient attention and time.

> QUEEN:
> Good Hamlet, cast thy nighted colour off
> And let thine eye look like a friend on Denmark.
> Do not for ever with thy vailed lids
> Seek for thy noble father in the dust.
>
> (1.2, 67–70)[2]

Hamlet's mother is asking him to change the direction of his gaze from his preoccupation with his dead father, towards the living, which includes his mother, his country, and the new King. She tries to reassure him that death is common:

> Thou know'st 'tis common, all that live must die,
> Passing through nature to eternity.
>
> (1.2, 71–72)

Hamlet replies,

> HAMLET:
> Ay, madam, it is common.
> QUEEN:
> If it be,

2 The quotations are taken from the Project Gutenberg eBook of *Hamlet* by William Shakespeare (1998).

Why seems it so particular with thee?
HAMLET:
Seems, madam! nay, it is; I know not seems.
'Tis not alone my inky cloak, good mother,
Nor customary suits of solemn black,
... Nor the dejected 'haviour of the visage,
... these indeed 'seem',
For they are actions that a man might play:
But I have that within which passeth show;
These but the trappings and the suits of woe.
(1.2, 74–86)

In this he claims a true grief within himself and accuses his 'good mother' of shallow feelings. Claudius joins Gertrude to admonish Hamlet.

KING:
'Tis sweet and commendable in your nature, Hamlet,
To give these mourning duties to your father:
But you must know, your father lost a father,
That father lost, lost his ...
... But to persever
In obstinate condolement is a course
Of impious stubbornness ...
... Fie! 'tis a fault to heaven,
A fault against the dead ...
(1.2, 87–102)

These are cogent arguments demanding that we mourn for a time and then move on, but Hamlet views them as corrupt. Shakespeare persuades us to take Hamlet's side through his loving depiction of his loyalty to his father, but he also shows us how the hatred of his mother dwarfs everything else in these early scenes, and how his grievance towards her diverts him from the task of mourning.

The Internal World of Melancholia

The opening lines of Hamlet's first great soliloquy later in the same scene are typically depressive and reflect his preoccupation with his inner world.

HAMLET:
O that this too too solid flesh would melt,
Thaw, and resolve itself into a dew!
Or that the Everlasting had not fix'd
His canon 'gainst self-slaughter.
(1.2, 129–132)

Hamlet longs for something hard inside him to soften or, if this proves to be impossible, to free himself from the pain of loss through suicide, if only it were not forbidden. He then proceeds to describe his despair.

> O God! O God!
> How weary, stale, flat, and unprofitable
> Seem to me all the uses of this world!
> Fie on't! O fie! 'tis an unweeded garden,
> That grows to seed; things rank and gross in nature
> Possess it merely.
>
> (1.2. 132–137)

Such depressive thoughts are typically seen in the early stages of mourning, and of course even more in melancholia, in which the flat, stale, and unprofitable world reflects the internal and external situations, both of which have lost all interest and value. Suddenly, however, Hamlet's mood changes and his thoughts come to life as he embarks on a passionate expression of outrage against his mother and stepfather. Grief turns to grievance in a righteous indignation that will dominate Hamlet through much of the play.

> That it should come to this!
> But two months dead: nay, not so much, not two:
> So excellent a king; that was, to this,
> Hyperion to a satyr …
> … And yet, within a month –
> Let me not think on't, – Frailty, thy name is Woman!
> … Why she, even she –
> O, God! a beast, that wants discourse of reason,
> Would have mourn'd longer – married with my uncle,
> My father's brother, but no more like my father
> Than I to Hercules: within a month:
> Ere yet the salt of most unrighteous tears
> Had left the flushing in her galled eyes,
> She married. O, most wicked speed, to post
> With such dexterity to incestuous sheets!
> It is not nor it cannot come to good:
> But break, my heart; for I must hold my tongue..
>
> (1.2, 137–159)

'But two months dead' seems far too short a time, and Hamlet persuades us that for Claudius and Gertrude the turning point of mourning came too soon. We can imagine that this is how it feels to Hamlet, and how his grievance and the hatred it provokes hardens his heart. He is no longer looking inwards, and the wrongdoing that the mourner normally accepts responsibility for is attributed to others. Mourning is stalled as guilt is externalised.

Remember Me: The Uncanny Power of Ghosts

Hamlet's indignant grievance is reinforced in the dramatic meeting with his father, who appears on the ramparts of the castle and reveals that his death was not an accident as claimed, but a murder that must be avenged. Hamlet immediately interrupts the work of mourning and throws himself fully behind the revenge.

He does this against his better judgement, knowing that ghosts are not supposed to return from the dead. Addressing the ghost, he asks:

O, answer me!
... Why thy canonized bones, hearsed in death,
Have burst their cerements; why the sepulchre,
Wherein we saw thee quietly inurn'd,
Hath oped his ponderous and marble jaws,
To cast thee up again.

(1.4, 26–32)

Hamlet was at the funeral and saw his father buried, so knows there was no ordinary or natural way he could appear alive. He should not be able to report from an afterlife that Hamlet knew as an

... undiscover'd country from whose bourn
No traveller returns[.]

(3.1, 85–86)

The ghost not only reveals the details of his own murder but describes what it is like to be confined in purgatory.

GHOST:
I am thy father's spirit,
Doom'd for a certain term to walk the night,
And for the day confined to fast in fires,
Till the foul crimes done in my days of nature
Are burnt and purged away.

(1.5, 13–17)

But hard on this comes the accusation that certain foul crimes have been done to him rather than by him.

GHOST:
...List, list, O list!
If thou didst ever thy dear father love –
... Revenge his foul and most unnatural murder.

(1.5, 26–29)

The ghost mentions but then ignores the foul crimes he himself has committed, for which he suffers in purgatory, and for which he needs to accept responsibility and guilt in order to be allowed to move on. Instead, he finds relief by attributing blame to someone outside the self, in this case Claudius, which leaves Hamlet facing a similar dilemma. Should he obey his father and join him in the demand for revenge, thereby also locating the guilt outside his father and outside himself? Or should he defy him, accepting that his father is dead so that he can face the task of mourning that he has embarked upon?[3]

The ghost is powerfully persuasive, and the bonds of respect, gratitude, and love are too strong to be severed. Hamlet ignores the possibility that the ghost is an evil spirit and, in complete identification with him, decides to devote his whole being to the pursuit of his commands.

> HAMLET:
> Haste me to know't, that I, with wings as swift
> As meditation or the thoughts of love
> May sweep to my revenge.
>
> (1.5, 33–35)

The ghost approves:

> GHOST:
> I find thee apt;
> And duller shouldst thou be than the fat weed
> That roots itself in ease on Lethe wharf
> Wouldst thou not stir in this.
>
> (1.5, 36–39)

The fat weed in ease on Lethe wharf reminds us of the unweeded garden in Hamlet's inner world, and the ghost suggests that if he does not act, he will sink into depression. The ghost finally binds Hamlet to him with the famous demand, 'Remember me', that will delay the progress of his mourning and keep him occupied with his father, at least until the revenge has been accomplished.

Hamlet replies:

> Remember thee?
> Ay, thou poor ghost, while memory holds a seat
> In this distracted globe. Remember thee?

3 Contact with the world of spirits and ghosts, and the idea of purgatory itself, were viewed as Catholic heresies in Protestant England, which leads Greenblatt (2001) to ask how they were able to appear in a Protestant play.

Yea, from the table of my memory
I'll wipe away all trivial fond records,
All saws of books, all forms, all pressures past,
That youth and observation copied there;
And thy commandment all alone shall live
Within the book and volume of my brain,
Unmix'd with baser matter.

(1.5, 100–109)

To enact the revenge demanded of him and to avoid any weakening of his resolve Hamlet swears that he will empty everything from his mind except the memory of his father. He does not think of himself, nor his future with Ophelia: he has not the slightest concern with politics, makes light of the threat of war, and has no ambition to become King himself.[4] The only proper subject of his thoughts must be revenge, and with this task he solidifies his link with his father and the past, and discards all concern for the future and for his own needs. Everything that might be creative in himself is postponed as he joins his father and puts his life on hold.[5] There is no question of letting go of the old and turning to the new until his revenge has been carried out. A similar conclusion is reached by Reisner (2019) in a paper that explores *Hamlet* and concludes that in his submission to his father he empties out his character.

The Demarcation between the Living and the Dead

We have seen how the ghost of Hamlet's father escapes from his tomb and, against all the laws of logic and religion, returns to haunt the living. He occupies that uncanny position neither fully dead nor yet still alive, and his arrival on the ramparts suggests to Hamlet that he has escaped from his grave because he has not been properly buried. This enables us to use Shakespeare's account to explore the importance of burial in helping us to accept the reality and irreversibility of death. It allows a separation of the concrete from the symbolic, as part of the separation between the body that is buried and the spirit that is

4 That Hamlet has been passed over in the succession to the throne is only mentioned once in the play, even though at the time *Hamlet* was written, the successor to Queen Elizabeth was a vital issue. On that one occasion he does refer to Claudius as:

He that hath killed my king and whored my mother,
Popped in between th' election and my hopes,
Thrown out his angle for my proper life …

(5.2, 69–71)

5 The contrast to the attitude of Cordelia in *King Lear* is striking. She is willing to give her father only what is his due, reserving part of her love for herself and the future.

liberated. This is emphasised in the Book of Common Prayer of 1549, where the priest recites,

> I commend thy soule to God the father almighty, and thy body to the grounde, earth to earth, asshes to asshes, dust to dust.[6]

The theme is explored in the graveyard scene, in which we can see the enormous difference between Hamlet's experience of his ghostly father, whose living presence continues to haunt him, and his memories of Yorick, the former court jester, who remains in his mind as a memory and a symbol of a person whose existence is firmly located in the past.

Hamlet exchanges witticisms with the Gravedigger, which come to centre on a famous skull that has lain in the earth some three and twenty years and turns out to be that of the King's jester.

> Alas, poor Yorick. I knew him, Horatio, a fellow of infinite jest, of most excellent fancy. He hath borne me on his back a thousand times; and now, how abhorred in my imagination it is! My gorge rises at it. Here hung those lips that I have kiss'd I know not how oft. Where be your gibes now? your gambols? your songs? your flashes of merriment, that were wont to set the table on a roar?
>
> (5.1, 141–145)

The descriptions of Yorick touch on happy times, but are also sad and, in contrast to the ghost, no longer indicate a concrete presence. The scene is abhorrent in Hamlet's imagination. Yorick has become a memory and a symbol as Hamlet recalls the lips that no longer hang from the jaw because the flesh has rotted away. The difference between Yorick and the Ghost seems to be just that difference between an object that has been accepted as dead and functions as a symbol to one that is still alive in the mind and persecutes the mourner with his demands. The importance of burial reminds us of the stench of decay and the risk of disease that persuade us that the dead must be put safely under the ground. There they must remain to confirm that the dead are really dead and out of reach of the living.

In contrast to his 'terrifying inwardness' (Bloom, 1999), Hamlet at times adopts an 'antic disposition', an ironic mood that puts everyone on edge and provides a kind of manic respite from the grief of mourning. In the exchanges that follow the precipitate murder of Polonius, Hamlet's wit plays with the distinction between the body and the spirit.

> KING:
> Now, Hamlet, where's Polonius?

6 The Ordre for the Buriall of the Dead. *The Book of Common Prayer* (1549), http://justus.anglican.org/resources/bcp/1549/BCP_1549.htm

> HAMLET:
> At supper.
> KING:
> At supper! Where?
> HAMLET:
> Not where he eats, but where he is eaten: a certain convocation of politic worms are e'en at him.
> ...
> KING:
> Where is Polonius?
> HAMLET:
> In heaven. Send thither to see. If your messenger find him not there, seek him i' th' other place yourself. But indeed, if you find him not within this month, you shall nose him as you go up the stairs into the lobby.
>
> (4.3, 18–34)

Hamlet in one breath accepts the spiritual passage of Polonius to either Heaven or Hell, but in the next breath locates his body through the stench of decay. However, when we get to the graveyard scene, time has passed and the remains of Yorick are no longer offensive. The work of mourning has buried the body but retained contact with the spirit. The distinction seems to weaken Hamlet's preoccupation with his father, and he gradually begins to pay attention to his own future.

Claudius and Hamlet realise that they are dangerous adversaries obliged to kill or be killed, and Hamlet's wish to kill Claudius becomes more a matter of survival than revenge. Gradually his preoccupation with his father has given way to a wish for his own life to be preserved, as he comes to value his life more and to value his father's honour less.[7] This seems to be a step in the recognition that his father is actually dead and no longer restorable. All that can be done is to allow him to be properly returned to the grave to become an ancestor.

7 Shakespeare has already ridiculed the value of honour in Falstaff's famous speech from *Henry IV, Part 1*:

> FALSTAFF:
> Can honour set to a leg? No. Or an arm? No. Or take away the grief of a wound? No. Honour hath no skill in surgery then? No. What is honour? A word. What is in that word, 'honour'? What is that 'honour'? Air. A trim reckoning! Who hath it? He that died o' Wednesday. Doth he feel it? No. Doth he hear it? No. 'Tis insensible, then? Yea, to the dead. But will it not live with the living?
> No. Why? Detraction will not suffer it. Therefore I'll none of it. Honour is a mere scutcheon. And so
> ends my catechism
>
> (5.1, 130–136)

The Heroic and the Human

There are some indications, too, that the ghost would be relieved if he could return to the grave. This is suggested by Loewald, when he says,

> Those who know ghosts tell us that they long to be released from their ghost-life and led to rest as ancestors.
>
> (1960, p. 29)

But neither Hamlet nor his father can let go of the need for revenge, and each is burdened by a grievance that they wish to be freed of. The internal situation is one where the individual feels that he cannot restore his damaged objects and put things right, but is also unable to escape from their demands.[8]

Hamlet clearly resents the fact that it is he who is expected to remedy the situation.

> The time is out of joint. O cursed spite,
> That ever I was born to set it right!
>
> (1.5, 205–206)

He wants to be free of the burden, and as we have seen, longs for something hard inside him to soften, as he cries

> O, that this too too solid flesh would melt,
> Thaw, and resolve itself into a dew!
>
> (1.2, 129–130)

But softness has its dangers, and makes Hamlet afraid that if he gave way to it he would melt into tears and lack the masculine strength necessary for revenge. When the ghost appears in the boudoir scene, usually played in his nightrobes rather than in armour, Hamlet pleads with him to avert his gaze for fear that it would make him weep.

> Do not look upon me
> Lest with this piteous action you convert
> My stern effects. Then what I have to do
> Will want true colour; tears perchance for blood.
>
> (3.4, 130–133)

To exchange the blood of revenge for the tears of sorrow is a betrayal of chivalric values and a move towards the human, which includes the acceptance of feminine elements that threaten Hamlet's much-needed masculinity. There

8 This has been referred to as the 'Joan Riviere dilemma' by Weiss (2020), namely, a situation where *'the individual can neither repair nor escape from his damaged internal objects'* (p. 1184; italics in the original).

follows a softening of his grievance against women in general, which releases the blocked feelings of love towards his mother and Ophelia. In the graveyard he is shocked to discover that Ophelia is dead and about to be buried in a suicide's grave. In his total devotion to his father he had emptied his mind of all thoughts of love, but they now return as he proclaims

> HAMLET:
> I lov'd Ophelia; forty thousand brothers
> Could not, with all their quantity of love,
> Make up my sum.
> (5.1, 224–226)

The awakening of his love has been made possible by the weakening of his identification with the military values held by the medieval knights which his father personified. When the Ghost appears on the ramparts, he is clad in the full armour that he wore when he defeated Old Fortinbras thirty years earlier, and now that Young Fortinbras threatens to invade and avenge the defeat of his father, the young Hamlet is expected to adopt a similar military role. But this is not in his character. He feels obliged to put things right and he fails; not because he is a coward, although he accuses himself of this, but because he questions the chivalric values pertaining to honour. He seems to move from an idealisation of phallic masculinity to one which values and respects femininity. This means that his masculinity is less phallic and more like the 'penis as link' described by Birksted-Breen (1996).

His willingness to think about the consequences of war and to imagine the cost of violent action is revealed in a chance encounter with a captain from the Norwegian army as it passes through Denmark. He learns that at Claudius' request, Young Fortinbras is going to spare Denmark but do battle over an insignificant part of Poland.

> a little patch of ground
> That hath in it no profit but the name.
> (4.4, 90–91)

And that

> Two thousand souls and twenty thousand ducats
> Will not debate the question of this straw!
> This is th' impostume of much wealth and peace,
> That inward breaks, and shows no cause without
> Why the man dies.
> (4.4, 97–101)

Here Hamlet recognises that the inhumanity of doing battle over honour and revenge functions as an 'impostume', that is, an abscess or cancer, that undermines the noble claims of chivalric values. Shapiro (2005) views this realisation as the turning point and darkest moment of the play. Even as he extols the need to fulfil his promise to avenge his father's reputation, Hamlet recognises the invisible rot that undermines these values.

His disgust over this corruption is repeated in the wonderfully dour soliloquy,

> How all occasions do inform against me,
> And spur my dull revenge.
>
> (4.4, 105–106)

Here we are shown an image of Fortinbras marching through Denmark on his way to slaughter Poles for a prize of war of no more value than an eggshell:

> Even for an eggshell. Rightly to be great
> Is not to stir without great argument,
> But greatly to find quarrel in a straw
> When honour's at the stake.
> ....
> ... while, to my shame, I see
> The imminent death of twenty thousand men
> That, for a fantasy and trick of fame,
> Go to their graves like beds, fight for a plot
> Whereon the numbers cannot try the cause,
> Which is not tomb enough and continent
> To hide the slain?
>
> (4.4, 126–138)

There is not even enough land gained to bury those who will be killed in the battle; yet he has to use the importance of honour to bolster his determination for revenge, and he insists that

> [O,] from this time forth
> My thoughts be bloody or be nothing worth.
>
> (4.4, 138–139)

Hamlet knows that he has to kill Claudius but cannot justify such an action, since the traditional avenger's appeal to honour rings hollow (Shapiro, 2005). He is now shifting his attention to his own future and fighting not for revenge but for survival, and for the survival of other values that we connect with being human.

Hamlet gives due weight to this when, as he dies, he names Fortinbras as his successor.

> I do prophesy th' election lights
> On Fortinbras. He has my dying voice.

> So tell him, with the occurrents more and less
> Which have solicited. The rest is silence. [Dies.]
>
> (5.2, 304–307)

I think Hamlet realises that a political leader needs to be able to defend the state and if necessary go to war, and that this is not the stuff that he is made of. As the stage is strewn with the poisoned bodies of the Danish royal household, we see the rot in the state of Denmark now being handed on to Fortinbras, as a successor who may have more of the military qualities that are needed to cleanse and defend it.

Mourning as a Tearing the Self Away from the Object

Perhaps the central question in mourning is how to extricate ourselves from the identification with the lost object. Freud saw the attachment as a form of narcissistic identification, 'I am the breast, the breast is me', or in this case 'I am my father, and I am as totally identified with his desires as if they were my own'. The identification results in a concrete, composite-object containing parts of the self. How then is it possible to dis-identify, to tear ourselves out of the object, to return the projected elements of the self to the ego and to allow the lost object to return to the grave? This means that we have to find the courage to defy and abandon the object and to consign him finally to a place in the past together with the dead.

One of the problems arises from the fact that the abandonment of the object can be felt as betrayal and as a murder. Anxiety and guilt are inevitable, and have to be tolerated if progress is to be made. This theme has been explored in relation to what Bloom (1973) refers to as 'the anxiety of influence', where writers fear their success will injure their predecessors. Britton has illustrated the same theme in psychoanalysts (1998), and I suspect that something similar contributed to the long delay before Darwin could publish the *Origin of the Species*. In a letter to J. D. Hooker (11 January 1844), he wrote:

> At last gleams of light have come, & I am almost convinced (quite contrary to opinion I started with) that species are not (it is like confessing a murder) immutable.
>
> (Darwin, 1844)

One can imagine the courage it took to defy the religious orthodoxy of his time; no doubt anxieties of a similar kind have been endured by every great innovator.[9]

9 Freud (1900a, p. 398) saw himself as this kind of rebel:

> ... not at all a man of science, not an observer, not an experimenter, not a thinker. I am by temperament nothing but a conquistador – an adventurer, if you want it translated – with all the curiosity, daring, and tenacity characteristic of a man of this sort.

The Dangers of Thinking

Hamlet repeatedly accuses himself of a failure to act and blames himself for turning to thought in place of action:

> Thus conscience does make cowards of us all,
> And thus the native hue of resolution
> Is sicklied o'er with the pale cast of thought,
> And enterprises of great pith and moment
> With this regard their currents turn awry,
> And lose the name of action.
>
> (3.1, 89–94)

For Hamlet, self-doubt interferes with the need to act. When he begins to think he becomes unsure of himself and, hesitating, he became weakened in his resolve. This is especially so in times of war; Hamlet is beginning to doubt the value of what he was fighting for and question the chivalric devotion to honour which demanded revenge for wrongs done to earlier generations. It is thinking that can lead to a rebellion against the dictates of duty on which the perpetuation of cycles of revenge depends. Such duty results from identifications with the ghosts of precursors and a failure to defy them and separate from their values.

In Freud's formulation of the dissolution of the Oedipus complex, we see the son submitting to the castration threat from his father and in compliance relinquishing his mother as his love object. This confirms the dominance of the father and creates a hierarchy in the family based on submission to threats. The identification, however, means that the son will in turn treat his progeny with the very same castration threats, and the cycle goes on until a son can rebel and defeat the father. I have suggested that Freud's model is a paranoid version of the Oedipus complex that perpetuates authoritarian rule through identification with the aggressor, and this contrasts with a depressive version that results when the son has the courage to defy the threat and stand up to the father. If the father is defeated, his death must be mourned and the associated burden of guilt carried (Steiner, 1996b, 2011a).

The Value and Necessity of Heroism and Revenge

Shakespeare, as always, offers both sides of any argument, and shows how courage is needed both to enact the revenge but also to refuse to do so. He accepts the existence of a situation where murder and revenge are right and necessary and need to be carried out but also one where it is proper to resist the demands made by vengeful internal objects that have returned from the dead to haunt us. It is as if Hamlet has to identify with the chivalric values of his father's age but also has to dis-identify with them to discover his own identity and find the courage to express it. Early in the mourning process, identification creates a strong link with the lost object, which is hyper-cathected (Freud,

1917b), but as mourning progresses the shift in attention at the turning point leads to an abandonment of the father and a move towards independence.

A Trust in Providence

Gradually Hamlet has loosened the bond to his father, rejecting the appeal to honour and barely mentioning revenge. He no longer feels obliged to solve the problems bequeathed to him, and most importantly, he is ready to face his own death. As he accepts the idea that some decisions can be left to providence, he is more able to respect the distinction between the human and the divine. The most significant difference between God and Man has to do with mortality, and to be fully human we must accept the inevitability of our own death. Indeed, if we consider that a vital achievement of mourning is to let the object go and admit we cannot keep it alive, then we are obliged to give up fantasies of our own immortality and the omnipotence that goes with it. This means that accepting our own death is an essential step in mourning, and helps us to move from concrete change to thinking symbolically. It is in the acceptance of his own death that Hamlet relinquishes possession of his object, and recognising his mortality allows providence to determine his fate.

> HAMLET:
> … There's a special providence in the fall of a sparrow. If it be, 'tis not to come; if it be not to come, it will be now; if it be not now, yet it will come. The readiness is all …
>
> (5.2, 151–152)

If life is to continue, we must be ready for it, and if it is death that we must face, then that too must be accepted. In his attempt to carry out his father's commands, Hamlet has been responsible for seven tragic deaths, which will shortly be followed by his own. He murdered Polonius, Rosenkranz, and Guildenstern; he drove Ophelia to suicide, and he was responsible for the deaths of Claudius, Gertrude, and Laertes, whose bodies now litter the stage. His longing to escape from the impossible demands imposed on him is at last granted by his own death, and since the royal succession is given over to Fortinbras, there is nothing more to say:

'The rest is silence'.

As part of the relinquishment of omnipotence, vengeance is also accepted as a divine rather than a human responsibility. This is summarised in the New Testament saying:

> Vengeance is mine;
> I will repay, saith the Lord.
> (King James Bible,
> Romans 12:19)

Perhaps the same is true of forgiveness, which Pope voiced so well in his famous couplet:

> To err is human;
> To forgive, divine
> (Alexander Pope,
> 1711, l. 525)

This consideration can also help us to accept that the wish for vengeance is part of human nature, and that it is naive to think we could rise above it and forgive our enemies.

This is expressed in a favourite quotation of Freud from Heinrich Heine: 'One must, it is true, forgive one's enemies – but not before they have been hanged.'[10]

Hamlet will not be returning as a ghost to haunt future generations with demands for revenge, but he remains in our minds as Shakespeare's most memorable character. He lives on as a symbol that can allow us to participate in the conflicts of the mourning process and to recognise the tragedy that the enactment of revenge inevitably gives rise to.

The play ends with a beautiful evocation of reconciliation and peace:

> HORATIO:
> Now cracks a noble heart.
> Good night, sweet prince,
> And flights of angels sing thee to thy rest.
> (5.2, 308–309)

10 A great imaginative writer may permit himself to give expression – jokingly, at all events – to psychological truths that are severely proscribed. Thus Heine confesses: 'Mine is a most peaceable disposition. My wishes are: a humble cottage with a thatched roof, but a good bed, good food, the freshest milk and butter, flowers before my window, and a few fine trees before my door; and if God wants to make my happiness complete, he will grant me the joy of seeing some six or seven of my enemies hanging from those trees. Before their death I shall, moved in my heart, forgive them all the wrong they did me in their lifetime. One must, it is true, forgive one's enemies – but not before they have been hanged.' Quote from Heine, *Gedanken und Einfälle* (Freud, 1930, p. 110).

4 Injury, Rage, Grievance, and Revenge in the Wrath of Achilles[1]

Introduction

In this chapter, a distinction is made between grievance and revenge. Both are expressions of the rage that arises in response to feelings of injustice and humiliation, but in revenge the rage is outwardly directed while in grievance it is held inwardly in a state of withdrawal. The difference is illustrated in an episode from the childhood of Coleridge but chiefly described in the origin and fate of the wrath of Achilles from Homer's *Iliad*. These examples allow me to argue that it may be necessary for rage to be expressed outwardly and openly for the damage it does to be fully recognised and for feelings of responsibility and guilt to be able to emerge. In order to be effective militarily in the heat of war, it may be necessary to deploy a paranoid defence against guilt which attributes all blame to the enemy. At the end of *The Iliad* the reconciliation between Achilles and Priam shows that mourning can be resumed when peace breaks out, and the factors that allow this are explored here and throughout the book.

The Importance of Grievance in Psychoanalysis

Confrontations involving grievance are an important obstacle to the progress of an analysis when they commonly interfere with the work of mourning. Instead of being relinquished and mourned, the lost object is installed in the ego, where an internal relationship of mutual disappointment develops. The internalised object functions as a critical super-ego to which the subject sometimes feels obliged to submit, and sometimes to rebel against.

For progress to be resumed, the object must be relinquished and mourned, and the process is blocked if grievance dominates. This is particularly likely to happen if the loss is felt to arise from an injury which inflicts a trauma, sometimes felt to be so severe it is thought of as a catastrophe. An internal situation such as that described by Freud in 'Mourning and Melancholia'

1 Based on J. Steiner (2025a), Injury, Grievance, and Revenge, in the Wrath of Achilles, *The International Journal of Psychoanalysis*, 106, 784–798.

DOI: 10.4324/9781003726135-5

(1917b) is then established, which leads to a relationship of mutual recrimination between the self and the internalised lost object that binds them indissolubly. When these are relived in the transference, a power struggle between the patient and the analyst can create obstacles to development that seem impossible to resolve.

Nor is the situation limited to that which follows loss through bereavement. Every developmental advance involves relinquishing the old and familiar, and embracing the new. The idealised relationship with the mother must be given up, despite the trauma of the various stages involved in separation-individuation (Mahler, 1972). The vital loss is that of the idealised mother's love, which becomes a feature of losses such as those involved in weaning, in moving to a separate room, going to school, leaving home, and eventually facing the loss of parents through their inevitable death. In each of these situations the loss can either be accepted and mourned or treated as a trauma that must be resisted and defied. When it is felt to be premature or unjust, it gives rise to grievance instead of acceptance. Confrontations following injuries to pride and status such as those I will describe in this chapter may give rise to a virtual state of war between patient and analyst, in which submissive grievance may alternate with triumphant enactments of revenge.

Whether it is possible to resolve grievances and allow the work of mourning to resume is always difficult to judge. Sometimes analysts can lessen the propensity to be pulled into the confrontations if they can understand how painful the losses sustained in the course of development can be. They may also be helped if they recognises that not only does the external object have to be mourned, but after it has been internalised, the object must again be relinquished and be mourned a second time. It commonly seems easier to accept the loss of the object externally than to relinquish it once it has been internalised.

Klein believed that the chief obstacles to mourning are the emergence of hostility and triumph (Klein, 1940), and it is the evident suffering they create that makes the repeated enactments of grievance and revenge seem so futile. However, the suffering associated with loss may be felt as even more unbearable. In her descriptions of the depressive position, Klein puts this in terms of realising that the object we love is the same as that which is so bitterly hated, and Riviere has movingly spelled out the agonies that arise when we feel impelled to repair our lost objects and do not have the capacity to do so.

> The content of the depressive position (as Melanie Klein has shown) is the situation in which all one's loved ones within are dead and destroyed, all goodness is dispersed, lost, in fragments, wasted and scattered to the winds; nothing is left within but utter desolation. Love brings sorrow, and sorrow brings guilt; the intolerable tension mounts, there is no escape, one is utterly alone, there is no one to share or help. (Riviere, 1936, p. 313)

In this chapter I will try to spell out how injuries to pride can produce a rage which can either be held internally as a grievance or expressed outwardly in the form of revenge. Part of the difficulty for the analyst in these situations arises from helplessness to alter the course of events, and sometimes all the analyst can do is try to understand the inevitable enactments in which grievances arise in the analysis.

Before proceeding to Homer's violent war epic, I will illustrate how grievance and revenge may arise in a more ordinary domestic quarrel between siblings by using an example from Richard Holmes' biography of Coleridge (2005):

> In the autumn of 1779, when he was seven, a quarrel took place between Sam and Frank [his older brother] which throws much light on the psychology of the youngest son, and which Coleridge himself shrewdly presented as a formative event. … It began … in the kitchen of the Vicarage, in a dispute about food – and favouritism. Sam, typically demanding, had asked his mother to prepare him some special sliced cheese for toasting. Frank stole in, and minced it up 'to disappoint the favourite', and a violent fight ensued. Fifteen years later Coleridge still entered into the drama as he wrote.
>
>> I returned, saw the exploit, and in an agony of passion flew at Frank – he pretended to have been seriously hurt by my blow, flung himself on the ground, and there lay with outstretched limbs – I hung over him moaning & in a great fright – he leaped up, & with a horse-laugh gave me a severe blow in the face – I seized a knife, and was running at him, when my Mother came in and took me by the arm – I expected a flogging – & struggling from her I ran away, to a hill at the bottom of which the Otter flows – about one mile from Ottery. …
>
> Sam fled … to his old friend the river, … and he remained there for the entire night … He said his prayers, and thought '*at the same time* with inward & gloomy satisfaction, how miserable my Mother must be!' …
>
> His mother, indeed, was 'almost distracted'. … half the town had turned out to search for the missing child … and 'no one went to bed'. At five in the morning Sam awoke, now frozen through, and too weak to move … [His cries were by good luck heard by a neighbour, who carried him in his arms to his father]
>
> 'I remember, & never shall forget, my father's face … and the tears stealing down … My Mother, as you may suppose, was outrageous with joy…'.
>
> Coleridge added that 'neither Philosophy or Religion' would allow him to forgive a local lady who suggested that he should have been whipped for this exploit. (Holmes, 2005, pp. 16–17)

Initially Coleridge was ready to enact a revenge in his attack with the knife, but this was prevented by the appearance of his mother and led to his withdrawal into a hiding place where he spent the night and nursed his grievance.

Such murderous feelings between siblings have been described by Juliet Mitchell (2013), who suggests that they emerge, even in normal families, when the family equilibrium is disturbed. The murderous rage is produced in response to an injury in which the infant feels dethroned from a privileged position by the loss of the mother's attention, typically by the arrival of the next baby. This rage would lead to actual murder if it were not for what Mitchell calls the *law of the mother*, comparable to Lacan's *law of the father*. This law enables the mother to intervene and prevent bloodshed in cases of sibling rivalry, as we saw in the case of Coleridge. However, from the point of view of the child, the law of the mother represents a betrayal of her promise of idealised union. Two objects of hatred then emerge: the brother with whom the war is waged and the mother who betrayed him by making room for his brother in the family. As we saw, Coleridge's withdrawal to his hiding place by the river was chiefly to hurt his beloved mother.

Coleridge ended up nursing his grievance and gaining satisfaction from the knowledge of the distress he was causing, being prepared to risk his life in order to torture his mother. That it was a beloved figure whom he tortured supports Mitchell's (2013) observation that the object is both adored and hated, and this is also commonly true of the sibling, who can be a valued ally as well as a rival (Davies, 2018). In the case of Coleridge, the grievance was not forgotten, and even 15 years later he could re-enter the drama as if it had just happened.

It is important, perhaps, to realise that Sam had to be found by the neighbour, as if he could not overcome the grievance of his own accord. In a similar way it may be necessary for the analyst to find their patient, and to recognise that the patient is unable to make the first move despite their longing for a reconciliation.

Because the object is both loved and hated, the attacks on it are meant to torture and threaten in order to force it to relent and, admitting the wrong, revert to the idealised relationship. When the child sees that their hatred has caused damage and even death, they have to face a guilt that may be enormous and perhaps unbearable. In fact, guilt played a large part in Coleridge's personality and played a role in both the mania and depression which he suffered throughout his life. His guilt was probably increased when, some two years after the fight, Frank departed for a career in the Navy and their father, after seeing him off, developed a fever and died. Then, to cap it all, Frank committed suicide by shooting himself in a fever in India at the age of 22.

The Trojan War

I will now turn to Homer's *Iliad* to look at the responses of Achilles which, on the grander stage of epic war poetry, seem to me to display feelings not so different from those of Coleridge.[2] First, a brief reminder that the war involved a ten-year siege of the city of Troy, a campaign which was itself a response to a humiliation and driven by a desire for vengeance. Under the leadership of Agamemnon, a coalition of Greek forces set out to avenge the dishonour done to his brother Menelaus, whose wife Helen had been abducted by Paris and taken to Troy. Heroes, such as Hector, Odysseus, Nestor, and Ajax, have important roles, but the pre-eminent character is Achilles, whose rage is a response to injuries done to him. In the tragic end of the siege, Troy was sacked, its menfolk slaughtered, and its women taken into slavery, but even for the victors, the whole venture was imbued with tragedy, extreme suffering, and innumerable deaths. *The Iliad* actually covers a period of less than two weeks in the tenth year of the war, and concentrates on events surrounding the wrath of Achilles.

The Wrath of Achilles

Achilles suffers two crushing injuries: first is his humiliation by his commander in chief Agamemnon, over his slave girl, Briseis. This injury leads to an impulse to kill Agamemnon, which is inhibited and replaced by a withdrawal into grievance. The second injury comes with the death of Achilles' friend, Patroclus, who had entered the battle in Achilles' place and is killed by his arch-enemy, the Trojan hero, Hector. This injury brings an end to the withdrawal and leads to an outburst of violence that cuts a path of devastation through the Trojan ranks and leads ultimately to the killing of Hector.

The famous opening stanza of the poem makes clear that Homer will focus on rage, both its murderous violence and its tragic consequences; in this case, the fact that countless Greeks were killed.

> Sing, goddess, the anger[3] of Peleus' son Achilleus and its devastation, which put pains thousandfold upon the Achaians, hurled in their multitudes to the house of Hades strong souls of heroes, but gave their bodies to be the delicate feasting of dogs, of all birds, and the will of Zeus was accomplished.
>
> (Book 1, p. 75)[4]

The First Injury: The Theft of the Slave Girl

Achilles is humiliated when his slave girl, Briseis, is taken from him by Agamemnon as an expression of his superior rank, and in response to this

2 I borrow these depictions of Achilles and Coleridge not to add to the field of literary theory, but in order to illustrate the role of grievance and revenge in the work of mourning and its obstacles.

3 In some translations the anger is described as 'wrath', which conveys the godlike status held by Achilles.

4 Quotations from *The Iliad* are taken from Homer, *The Iliad*, translated by Richard Lattimore (University of Chicago Press, Kindle Edition, 2011).

injury he withdraws in pique, refusing to fight and producing a massive defeat for the Greeks as a consequence.

Briseis was a prize of war won when her city, adjacent to Troy, was sacked, and for Achilles, she was a trophy whose loss was viewed as a humiliation. Agamemnon himself has been forced to return his concubine to her father in order to avert Apollo's punishment in the form of a plague, and his taking of Briseis is also a response to humiliation. Both have felt their pride wounded and they clash in a confrontation over power, in which Agamemnon threatens to take back the slave girl by force and Achilles threatens to withdraw and even to sail back to his home.

> O wrapped in shamelessness, with your mind forever on profit,
> how shall any one of the Achaians readily obey you
> either to go on a journey or to fight men strongly in battle?
> I for my part did not come here for the sake of the Trojan spearmen
> to fight against them, since to me they have done nothing.
> Never yet have they driven away my cattle or my horses,
> never in Phthia where the soil is rich and men grow great did they spoil my harvest ...
>
> (Book 1, p. 79)

In this speech Achilles claims that he had nothing against the Trojans and only took part in the war as a favour to Agamemnon, whose brother Menelaus had been humiliated by the abduction of Helen. In his view, the whole war had no purpose other than to defend Agamemnon's pride.

In response to these insults, Agamemnon uses his rank to force Achilles to submit.

> Not so quickly, brave as you are, godlike Achilles –
> trying to cheat me. Oh no, you won't get past me, ...
> What do you want? To cling to your own prize
> while I sit calmly by – empty-handed here? ...
> ....
> I will be there in person at your tents to take Briseis
> in all her beauty, your own prize –
> so you can learn just how much greater I am than you.
>
> (Book 1, p. 80)

In response to this claim of superiority, the wrath of Achilles mounts; it is briefly directed outwards as he draws his sword, but is quickly inhibited through the intervention of the goddess Athena, rather as Coleridge was pulled back by his mother.

> So he spoke. And the anger came on
> Peleus' son, and within his shaggy breast the heart

> was divided two ways, pondering whether to draw
> from beside his thigh the sharp sword, driving away all those who stood between and kill the son of Atreus, or else to check the spleen within and keep down his anger.
> Now as he weighed in mind and spirit these two courses and was drawing from its scabbard the great sword, Athene descended from the sky. … [and] standing behind Peleus' son caught him by the fair hair, appearing to him only, for no man of the others saw her.
>
> (Book 1, p. 80)

He puts away his sword but continues to mount verbal attacks and to assert his intention to withdraw from the war. Eventually he claims that in his absence, the defeats to be inflicted on the Greeks will be so terrible that Agamemnon will be sorry for what he has done and will 'eat his heart out'.

> And this shall be a great oath before you:
> some day longing for Achilleus will come to the sons of the Achaians, all of them. Then stricken at heart though you be, you will be able to do nothing, when in their numbers before manslaughtering Hektor they drop and die.
> And then you will eat out the heart within you in sorrow,
> that you did no honour to the best of the Achaians.
>
> (Book 1, p. 81)

After the confrontation in which Achilles confirms his withdrawal, he seeks out his mother, the sea goddess Thetis, and gives her his version of the wrongs done to him. Unlike Coleridge's mother, Thetis fails to endorse *the law of the mother* and instead she takes his side, viewing Achilles as the wronged infant and justifying revenge. With the help of Zeus, the Trojans gain a temporary victory, which is to turn the tide of the war against the Greeks. Despite the terrible slaughter of his compatriots, Achilles refuses to relent and, regardless of the apologies and gifts from Agamemnon and pleas from the other Greek leaders, he remains adamant and refuses to fight. He seems to feel no guilt over the slaughter of his compatriots and remains caught up in the justification of his grievance.

The Second Injury: The Death of Patroclus.

A complete turnaround takes place when Achilles' adored friend Patroclus is killed, and this second injury seems to reverse the direction of his rage, provoking an outwardly directed violence of enormous ferocity and cruelty. The first injury is especially one to his pride, but the second injury is more substantial because his friend Patroclus is dead and in normal circumstances would have been buried and mourned. Instead, Achilles gives priority to revenge and the loss cannot be attended to and mourned until a pause in the fighting can be found.

Earlier, Patroclus returns from a survey of the battlefield, weeping in his concern for the suffering of the Greeks caused by Achilles' withdrawal.

> ... [He] stood by him and wept warm tears, like a spring dark-running that down the face of a rock impassable drips its dim water;

But Achilles is unmoved and mocks him.

> Why then are you crying like some poor little girl, Patroklos, who runs after her mother and begs to be picked up and carried, and clings to her dress, and holds her back when she tries to hurry, and gazes tearfully into her face, until she is picked up? You are like such a one, Patroklos, dropping these soft tears.

Patroclus explains that his tears were in response to the suffering of the Greeks.

> Son of Peleus, far greatest of the Achaians, Achilleus, do not be angry; such grief has fallen upon the Achaians. For all those who were before the bravest in battle are lying up among the ships with arrow or spear wounds.
>
> (Book 16, p. 351)

Patroclus is the kindest figure in Achilles' camp, showing concern for those suffering from the cruelty of war and offering care to Briseis and the other slaves. He seems to represent a more humane side of Achilles, but one that is seen as effeminate and unacceptable in a warrior. Achilles seems particularly afraid of harbouring any feelings of softness, regret, or sorrow, even though he himself runs to cry to his mother when he feels wronged. Perhaps to engage in the brutality of war he had to repudiate his femininity (Freud, 1937), and it is only towards the end of the poem, as we shall see, that he is able to relent and to weep when he meets Priam.

Achilles is untouched by the pleading of Patroclus, and has no regard for the suffering of the Greeks because he remains trapped in his grievance over his slave girl.

> ... but this thought comes as a bitter sorrow to my heart ... that the girl ... the Achaians chose out for my honor, ... is taken back out of my hands by powerful Agamemnon, the son of Atreus, as if I were some dishonoured vagabond.
>
> (Book 16, p. 352)

Eventually Achilles is persuaded by Patroclus to allow him to enter the battle in his place, where, disguised in his armour, he might stand in for Achilles.

Patroclus goes on to fight bravely, but is eventually confronted by Hector and killed. The terrible news is brought to Achilles by a messenger:

> Ah me, son of valiant Peleus; you must hear from me the ghastly message of a thing I wish never had happened. Patroklos has fallen, and now they are fighting over his body which is naked. Hektor of the shining helm has taken his armor.

Achilles is bereft.

> He spoke, and the black cloud of sorrow closed on Achilleus. In both hands he caught up the grimy dust, and poured it over his head and face, and fouled his handsome countenance, and the black ashes were scattered over his immortal tunic. And he himself, mightily in his might, in the dust lay at length, and took and tore at his hair with his hands, and defiled it.
>
> (Book 18, pp. 396–397)

It is this second injury that, added to the first, provoked the violent revenge in which Achilles returns to the battlefield with renewed hatred that is now directed outwards. In other circumstances his grief in the course of mourning his friend might have led to feelings of responsibility and guilt, but any such feelings are interrupted by a rage that takes him over completely. The immediate outcome is that Patroclus lies unburied and un-mourned while Achilles acts to avenge him.

> Food and drink mean nothing to my heart but blood does, and slaughter, and the groaning of men in the hard work.
>
> (Book 18, pp. 419–420)

Achilles' Revenge: The Debacle of Slaughter without Restraint

One of the striking features of *The Iliad* is the detailed depiction of the terrifying violence of war. We, the audience, are horrified by the graphic descriptions given to us by Homer, but we are also struck by the fact that Achilles, while observing the bloodshed, is only driven on to more cruelty, as if consumed with bloodlust. Here are some examples of the violence:

> … now Tros with his hands was reaching
>
> for the knees, bent on supplication, but [Achilles] stabbed with his sword at the liver so that the liver was torn from its place, and from it the black blood drenched the fold of his tunic and his eyes were shrouded in darkness as the life went.

> Next from close in he thrust at Moulios with the pike at the ear, so the bronze spearhead pushed through and came out at the other ear.
>
> … so before great-hearted Achilleus the single-foot horses trampled alike dead men and the axle under the chariot was all splashed with blood. … and the son of Peleus was straining to win glory, his invincible hands spattered with bloody filth.
>
> (Book 20, pp. 438–439)

The Death of Hector

The final target of Achilles' revenge is the Trojan hero, Hector, hated even more as the killer of Patroclus. However, even the killing of Hector does not assuage his rage, which is further expressed when he desecrates Hector's body by dragging it round the walls of Troy in full view of Hector's family.

> He spoke, and now thought of shameful treatment for glorious Hektor. In both of his feet at the back he made holes by the tendons in the space between ankle and heel, and drew thongs of ox-hide through them, and fastened them to the chariot so as to let the head drag, and mounted the chariot, and lifted the glorious armor inside it, then whipped the horses to a run, and they winged their way unreluctant. A cloud of dust rose where Hektor was dragged, his dark hair was falling about him, and all that head that was once so handsome was tumbled in the dust.
>
> (Book 21, p. 468)

The Funeral of Patroclus

Returning to his camp, Achilles has an elaborate funeral pyre built for Patroclus. He seems to have found a kind of peace through the enactment of his revenge, of which he is proud and which is admired by his fellow Greeks. Something seems to have been worked through, as if the violence is an achievement that has brought justice and undone the wrong that has been inflicted. Finally, he does see to the cremation of Patroclus, which allows him to begin to mourn the loss of his friend. But even so Achilles is not fully able to let him go. Knowing that his own death is imminent, he plans that their bones be buried together in two stone jars, side by side.

Achilles and Priam

In the final book of *The Iliad* we see a softening of Achilles' rage, which enables a move towards a reconciliation to take place. When Priam comes in person to the Greek camp seeking the body of Hector, his son, Achilles admires his courage and, looking on Priam with a new respect, listens attentively to his story. Priam describes the painful losses he has suffered, and reminds Achilles that his own father will one day die and will have to be mourned.

> 'Honor then the gods, Achilleus, and take pity upon me remembering your father, yet I am still more pitiful; I have gone through what no other mortal on earth has gone through; I put my lips to the hands of the man who has killed my children.'
>
> So he spoke, and stirred in the other a passion of grieving for his own father. He took the old man's hand and pushed him gently away, and the two remembered, as Priam sat huddled at the feet of Achilleus and wept close for manslaughtering Hektor and Achilleus wept now for his own father, now again for Patroklos.
>
> (Book 23, pp. 510–511)

The two men weep together and elicit pity and compassion for each other. Both are able to put their hatred to one side and for the first time Achilles allows human feeling to emerge as his rage lessens. His ability to weep seems to have been a factor that enables the loss to be mourned.

Even then the rage remains close to the surface, and Achilles warns Priam that it could easily explode once more. He continues to be sensitive to issues of honour and is even concerned that his mercy to Priam could be felt as a betrayal by the dead Patroclus from beyond the grave. It is perhaps significant that Achilles is sought and found by Priam just as the young Coleridge was found by his neighbour, again helping the analyst to understand that the patient may be too proud to make the first move.

The Funeral of Hector: The Trojans and the Greeks Compared

Priam returns to Troy with the body of his son and the poem ends with the funeral of Hector, which is markedly different from that of Patroclus. Throughout the drama, Trojans have been portrayed as more humane, more family-oriented, and less ruthless than the Greeks. They are, after all, *defending* their city, and remain in contact with their wives and mothers, whose survival they are responsible for. The Greeks by contrast are occupiers in a foreign land, far from their families, and living in a military camp where the only women are captive concubines.

In lieu of funereal games, the Trojans are preoccupied with their grief and with the praise of Hector, expressed with special anguish by the women: Hector's mother Hecuba, his sister Cassandra, and his wife Andromache.

> She spoke, and there was no man left there in all the city nor woman, but all were held in sorrow passing endurance. They met Priam beside the gates as he brought the dead in. First among them were Hektor's wife and his honored mother who tore their hair, and ran up beside the smooth-rolling

> wagon, and touched his head. And the multitude, wailing, stood there about them. And now and there in front of the gates they would have lamented all day till the sun went down and let fall their tears for Hektor.
>
> (Book 24, p. 516)

The Iliad ends with this funeral, but we know that Achilles is to be killed soon after and, when Troy is finally sacked, the violent revenge continues into the next generation. Achilles' son Neoptolemus, also known as Pyrrhus, savagely hacks Priam to death, takes Hector's wife Andromache as his slave, and dashes the body of his infant son against the city walls. Achilles is dead but his savagery lives on.

The Characteristics of Grievance: Injustice and Injury

I would like to emphasise two main features of grievance. First, that it consists of a rage that arises in response to an injury that is deemed to be unjust. Secondly, in grievance, the impulse to enact the revenge is inhibited and leads to a withdrawal where the revenge is expressed in phantasy rather than action (Hoggett, 2018; Feldman, 2008; Wurmser, 2009).

The sense of injustice is commonly so powerful that an all-or-nothing situation is established, where the victim is completely innocent and the wrongdoer completely guilty. Severe super-ego judgements dominate, and morality becomes so important that it is difficult to evaluate the rights and wrongs of the conflict. What *should* have happened is more important than what *did* happen, so that in the heat of the violence it becomes impossible to appeal to the subject's capacity for reflection and self-examination. This is a feature of the splitting that is characteristic in times of war, in which *we* are all good and *the enemy* is all bad. It indicates that the internal relationship between the injured and the injuring parties is on a war footing and hence implacable and unresolvable. The injustice is felt to involve an abuse of power and a loss of status that produces an unbearable humiliation in the victim. The humiliation calls for immediate relief, which is effectively achieved by a phantasy of triumphant revenge that reverses the shame through inflicting it on the other.

The Withholding of the Attack

It is the withdrawal of rage that differentiates grievance from revenge, and the result is a predominance of phantasy over action. In grievance, revenge is planned, imagined, and ruminated over in scenarios in which both the humiliation and its triumphant reversal are endlessly repeated. An up-and-down world is created consisting only of humiliation or triumph, in which one party or the other dominates for a time. It is these phantasies that keep subject and object bound together, held onto as long as the grievance is held onto. Feldman (2008) has pointed out that the nursing of grievance can become a source of perverse gratification, especially when it becomes erotised, and there certainly seems to be a special excitement when feelings of humiliation are transformed into those of triumph as the tables are turned on the hated object.

Reversing the wrong seems so wholly justified that the damage done by the withdrawal gives rise to no guilt and, because it is done only verbally and in phantasy, it can be magically undone. This happens despite the fact that the person's withdrawal and indirect expression of rage are intended to hurt the perpetrator and lead him to regret his actions and admit he was wrong. Coleridge found satisfaction in the thought of his mother's misery, while Achilles claims that Agamemnon will be 'stricken at heart' and regret that he injured 'the best of the Achaeans'. The victim is unaware that he himself has been cruel, but the observer is struck by the terrible consequences of the withdrawal. In the case of Coleridge, we realise how devastated his parents were, and in the case of Achilles we are faced with the appalling slaughter his withdrawal visits on his fellow Greeks. The absence of any awareness of guilt means that no feelings of regret or remorse can bring the cycle of attacks to a halt, and this gives grievance an unyielding quality.

The Garden of Eden Illusion

The grievances of adult life can be traced back to early infantile rebuffs such as those that arise when primitive phantasies of an idealised union with the mother are shattered. These Garden of Eden Illusions eventually collapse when the reality of the Oedipus situation leads to a terrible fall from the bliss of uniqueness into a lowly position of inferiority (Steiner, 2018). It is especially the mother's independence, made manifest when her thoughts turn elsewhere, that leads the infant to feel dropped and betrayed. These are universal experiences that inevitably lead to grievance, but it also commonly happens that grievance is amplified by traumatic events which face the infant with the fact that bad objects exist, from which the mother cannot always protect him. Much must depend on how the rage is dealt with, for example whether it is expressed openly as an attack or held back inwardly as a grievance.

The Characteristics of Revenge

In contrast to grievance, the active pursuit of revenge is an open expression of hatred that leads to tangible and visible consequences. In this way an opportunity arises that can enable some insight into the damage to be recognised even if it is not always heeded. Both revenge and grievance interfere with mourning. The injury has led to a loss, sometimes of an actual object through death, but sometimes as the loss of love, and with it comes the loss of the ideal that has sustained the illusion of perfection. For development to proceed these losses must be accepted and mourned, so that a turning point of mourning is reached in which the past is relinquished and attention shifts to the future (Steiner, 2023c).

Such moves are not possible when the rage is withheld in grievance, and even when it is expressed actively as revenge the process is difficult and the outcome uncertain. The opportunity to take stock is not always heeded, and the drive to revenge, as we have seen in the case of Achilles, may itself be unstoppable. In the throes of rage the subject may be in no state to observe, and if he is able to observe, he may not be able to respond to the damage his violence is doing. However, revenge, because it is open and generous, is more likely to lead to a stop than is the withdrawal into grievance. It may be, however, that it is only after revenge has been enacted and the damage viewed that that the loss can be accepted and mourned. This recalls again Heine's observation that one must forgive one's enemies, but not before they have been hanged (Freud, 1930, p. 110).

Qualities Needed in Times of War

The moral difficulty of acting out revenge that does real and evident damage means that heroic qualities are required to make the shift from grievance to revenge, and it is these qualities that are especially valued in times of war. It is then that a paranoid-schizoid mentality becomes more important than that of the depressive position. *The Iliad* is a war epic and to exact his revenge Achilles displays those heroic qualities that are so admired and lead to his renown. Courage, conviction, loyalty, self-sacrifice, strength, and ruthlessness are all of value in war, while there are no medals for kindness, self-doubt, regret, or concern for the enemy, which only seem to emerge in peacetime. Achilles is praised because of his fearless aggression, and it is only an observer such as the reader of *The Iliad* who, being outside the fray, can see that he is also shameless and apparently guilt-free, as he enacts his revenge. We are horrified at the violence and long for a truce, so that the killing can stop and mourning of the terrible losses can begin. In the analytic situation, the ability to shift from grievance to revenge requires similar heroic qualities, not only in the battles between patient and analyst but in the ability to stand up to a super-ego that forbids violence. There is, of course, no way to avoid guilt when revenge does such terrible damage, and it may then be necessary to live with guilt and to suffer its consequences.

It is perhaps only when peace is resumed that the capacity to think and evaluate the rights and wrongs of the grievance can emerge. The moral values of the super-ego may then have to be evaluated alongside the reality issues of the rights and wrongs of the injury (Britton, 2018). Sometimes the damage done by an open attack, however great and evident, may be less than the corrosive, long-term damage of withdrawal into grievance. It may then also become possible to see that the current grievance is a repetition of earlier injuries that have not been properly worked through. Of course, the pain of mourning will confront the mourner with such terrible guilt and remorse that is so difficult to bear that an escape back into grievance may be sought.

The Importance of a Double Loss

It seems generally to be the case that the full impact of a loss requires a kind of *après-coup* (deferred action, *Nachträglichkeit*), in the form of a second loss to make itself felt (Laplanche and Pontalis, 1967, p. 111). The initial loss of the external object is denied when it is installed internally, and a second, more devastating loss takes place when the internal object is relinquished and mourned.

The first loss for Achilles is a blow to his dignity when Briseis, his slave girl, is taken by Agamemnon. This is for Achilles chiefly a loss of pride since for him, Briseis is a trophy of war rather than a loved object. The second loss follows the death of Patroclus and involves not just a loss of pride but an actual loss of a dear and valued friend. This second loss means that his guilt towards his friend as well as to his fellow Greeks will have to be faced. No mourning is, however, allowed to take place until his revenge has been taken, and to ensure this Patroclus's funeral has to be delayed. It is only after the revenge has run its course and Patroclus has been buried that Achilles is able to soften his rage and permit a degree of reconciliation with Priam. It is such softening, often associated with tears, that enables a move towards the turning point of mourning to take place.

In a similar way, Coleridge engaged in a war within his family, and attacked his brother openly with murder in his heart. It was then that he was stopped by his mother, and this led him to turn his rage against her in his withdrawal. The violent revenge was prevented when his mother held him back, and a second, deeper wound was inflicted when she could no longer be thought of as his special ally because she also protected his brother. His rage then turned against his mother, and it was she who would suffer if he died.

Fear of a Breakdown that Has Already Happened

The fear of an open expression of revenge may be especially significant if the object has served as a protection against breakdown. Psychotic anxieties of disintegration are relieved if the fragments can be projected into an object, in a process which Bion has described as containment (1962). When this happens, the fear of breakdown is reduced in the presence of the object, which is installed internally and serves to avoid loss and breakdown. The threat of a second loss that involves the internal object being relinquished means that the fear of breakdown returns. I think this may be the basis of what Winnicott (1974) calls 'a fear of breakdown that has already happened'. The fear of breakdown can then be thought of as the fear of the loss of the illusion that the protective object continues to protect. Achilles had the consolation that when he died his glory would lead him to be remembered and thus confer a kind of immortality which may have helped him to display the courage and fortitude that made him a hero. However, the fact that his mother's magic, even in the form of his new armour, failed to protect Patroclus must have shattered the illusion of her omnipotence and of his own invincibility. Eventually his acceptance of his mortality enabled Achilles to bury Patroclus and prepare for his own death.

The Release of Love through the Enactment of Hatred

These considerations suggest that grievance reflects an internal state of war that delays a move to the depressive position and prevents the experience of guilt and the wish to make reparation. Without reparation, the horrors of revenge become unbearable, and this can only change if peace can be resumed after revenge has been enacted. We may be dealing here with an example of the release of love through the enactment of hatred, which Klein described in her *Lectures on Technique* (Steiner, 2017). She illustrates how feelings of sorrow can deepen the experience of love, but only when we recognise that we have hurt and injured our good objects. She writes

> I hold the view that … sorrow, guilt and anxiety are part and parcel of the complex relation to objects which we call love. It is from these conflicts that the drive to reparation springs, which is not only a powerful motive for sublimations, but also is inherent in feelings of love … (Klein, in Steiner, 2017, p. 12)

For this to happen, the hatred must be given voice, and grievance must change to revenge so that the suffering caused can be recognised and responded to. The feelings of remorse and guilt may then reveal the existence of a deeper love, which Klein believed helped the patient to make reparation and begin to restore their internal world. Such thoughts raise the possibility that a reconciliation between patient and analyst might emerge if the mutual hurt inflicted is made apparent, and that guilt, sorrow, and love are released in order to support a compromise. Experience seems to confirm that such hopes are naïve until a point has been reached when the struggle comes to a natural end. How and when this can happen remains poorly understood, but it seems that mourning cannot proceed as long as there is unfinished business to be resolved. Nevertheless, change, when it does happen, can be moving and life-changing, as it releases the capacity to mourn and to resume development.

5 Successful and Unsuccessful Mourning

Revisiting Klein[1]

Introduction

In this chapter I will examine two themes of central importance to our understanding of mourning. First, the question of what comprises the work of mourning, what is achieved when it is successful, and what the consequences are when it fails. Second, I will look at the obstacles that can arise which interfere with the work, and which result in a failure to mourn and, if prolonged, to the development of melancholia. Both these themes are explored in Klein's paper 'Mourning and its Relation to Manic-Depressive States' (Klein, 1940), and I begin by returning to this important paper, in which two cases, Mrs A and Mr B, are described. Mrs A's mourning was considered to have been successful despite important resistances, while Mr B's mourning was blocked, with serious consequences. The recent publication of *Klein's Lectures on Technique* (Steiner, 2017) and *Narrative of an Adult Analysis* (English, 2023) use material from the Klein Archives, and provide a fund of detailed clinical material about Mr B that I hope will enable the obstacles to mourning to be further explored.

Klein begins her paper on mourning by restating and elaborating several of Freud's classical findings from 'Mourning and Melancholia' (Freud, 1917b). She then describes two examples of mourning: Mrs A,who eventually was able to accept the death of her son and to face the reality of her loss, and Mr B, who was seriously depressed and whose mourning for his mother was blocked. Klein was concerned to illustrate the way a normal mourner can sever his attachment to the lost object and re-establish connections with the external world, and to contrast this with the melancholic, who is trapped in a preoccupation with the lost object that he is unable to relinquish.

1 This chapter has not been previously published. It is based on a paper given at the West Lodge Conference in London in 2024.

DOI: 10.4324/9781003726135-6

Mrs A: Normal Mourning

Mrs A's son is described as having died suddenly while at school, to which she reacted with shock, feeling shattered and numb. As she improved, she began sorting out her letters, keeping his and throwing others away, trying to 'keep him safe inside herself'. Klein sees this as an example of the way an object can be internalised to prevent the loss being registered. She also noted that, in the first week Mrs A did not cry much, and 'tears did not bring her the relief which they did later on' (1940, p. 138).

Hostility and Triumph as Obstacles to Mourning

Klein goes on to describe how Mrs A's hostility and triumph towards her son delayed the acceptance of her loss. This was expressed in a dream in which a mother dressed in black appeared with her son, who had died or was going to die. Instead of sorrow, Mrs A felt hostility to them both, and her associations brought up a childhood memory which Klein described in detail.

When Mrs A was a little girl, her brother, who had difficulties in his schoolwork, was going to be tutored by a schoolfellow of his own age (I will call him B). B's mother had come to see Mrs A's mother to arrange about the coaching, and Mrs A. remembered this incident with very strong feelings. B's mother behaved in a patronising way, and her own mother appeared to her to be rather dejected. She herself felt that a fearful disgrace had fallen upon her very much admired and beloved brother and the whole family. This brother, a few years older than herself, seemed to her full of knowledge, skill, and strength – a paragon of all the virtues – and her ideal was shattered when his deficiencies at school came to light.

At the same time, however, the death wishes against her own brother and the wish to inflict punishment and deprivation upon her own mother through the loss of her son (Mrs A's brother) – very deeply repressed wishes – were part of her dream thoughts. It now appeared that Mrs A, with all her admiration and love for her brother, had been jealous of him on various grounds, envying his greater knowledge, his mental and physical superiority, and also his possession of a penis.

> When her brother died, besides great sorrow, she unconsciously felt triumph over him, derived from her early jealousy and hatred, and [suffered] corresponding feelings of guilt. She had carried over some of her feelings for her brother into her relation to her son. ...The mourning for her brother, together with the sorrow, the triumph and the guilt experienced in relation to him, entered into her present grief, and was shown in the dream. (Klein, 1940, pp. 139–140)

These details allow us to surmise, in agreement with Grosskurth (1986), that Mrs A was a slightly disguised version of Klein herself. She had lost her son

Hans in a mountain accident in 1934 and had had an intense and idealised relationship with her brother Emanuel, who died in 1902, when Klein was 20.

Klein used her account of Mrs A to illustrate the way that, even in normal individuals, hostility and triumph can function to block mourning. In this she openly disagreed with Freud, who had not been able to observe triumph in normal mourning.

> At this point I find that my view differs from that of Freud … In my experience, feelings of triumph are inevitably bound up even with normal mourning and have the effect of retarding the work of mourning, or rather they contribute much to the difficulties and pain which the mourner experiences. (Klein, 1940, p. 137)

I think she wanted to show that problems with mourning are universal, and that hatred and triumph, while they threatened to block mourning in the case of Mrs A, were much more of an obstacle in the case of Mr B. In spite of the obstacles, and perhaps partly because she was able to become conscious of them, Mrs A was able to separate from her dead son and let him go.

The Acceptance of Loss: Separating the Living from the Dead

This relinquishment was described in the context of a dream:

> Two nights after [the first] dream she [Mrs A] dreamt again. She was flying with her son, and he disappeared. She felt that this meant his death – that he was drowned. She felt as if she, too, were to be drowned – but then she made an effort and drew away from the danger, back to life.
>
> The associations showed that in the dream she had decided that she would not die with her son but would survive. It appeared that even in the dream she felt that it was good to be alive and bad to be dead. In this dream the unconscious knowledge of her loss is much more accepted than in the one of two days earlier. Sorrow and guilt had drawn closer. (Klein, 1940, p. 141)

Here I think Klein felt supported by Freud when he wrote: 'Reality-testing has shown that the loved object no longer exists, and it proceeds to demand that all libido shall be withdrawn from its attachments to that object' (Freud, 1917b, p. 243).

It seems that it was her awareness of her love of life that led Mrs A to separate herself from her son. He was allowed to fall and die, while she pulled herself away in order to live. She severed her attachment, and in the process she withdrew her libido from the old relationship and enabled it to be invested in new objects. The direction of the libido was reversed; it was removed from her son, who now could be accepted as a figure from the past, and became free to be invested in the future.

Following this critical point in her mourning, Klein described how

> Mrs A found some comfort in looking at nicely situated houses in the country, and in wishing to have such a house of her own. But this comfort was soon interrupted by bouts of despair and sorrow. She now cried abundantly and found relief in tears. (Klein, 1940, p. 141)

The acceptance of separateness between the living Mrs A and her dead son was achieved through the heeding of what Freud called the verdict of reality. She was able to listen to this verdict because, to some extent at least, she had worked through her grievance in relation to the injury she felt when her son died. This injury revived the hostility she remembered feeling towards her brother, and she became aware of the pleasure she got from feelings of triumph towards her brother, her mother, and now her son. Triumph gave rise to guilt, which for a time was dealt with by projection, in what Klein called the paranoid defence against guilt. In the case of Mrs A, however, the feeling of humiliation and the hatred it provoked, the phantasies of triumph, and the guilt resulting from these, were at least to some extent able to be recognised and accepted, and it was this acceptance that enabled her hostility to be transformed into sorrow, as her son was recognised as gone.

Mr B: Mourning Blocked by Hostility and Triumph

Klein argued that, even in normal individuals, the early psychotic anxieties which are reactivated in mourning make it reasonable to view mourning as an illness resembling a manic-depressive state. These features are especially prominent when hostility comes to dominate and block the work of mourning.

The greatest danger for the mourner comes from the turning of his hatred against the lost loved person. One of the ways in which hatred expresses itself in the situation of mourning is in feelings of triumph over the dead person. Thus death, however shattering for other reasons, is to some extent also felt as a victory, and gives rise to triumph, and therefore all the more to guilt (Klein, 1940, p. 137).

Klein described how compared to Mrs A, the interference with mourning was more serious in the case of Mr B even though the emergence of hostility and triumph followed a similar pattern. In his case, she argued that the hostility became intense and intransigent because it arose in relation to a specific phantasy, namely that of the combined parents, who emerged as a source of great anxiety and hatred.

Mr B's Response to the Death of His Mother

When she turned to describing Mr B, Klein concentrated on a time when his mother was dying and his sessions became full of hatred and bitterness towards both his mother and Klein. He accused his mother of having made his father unhappy, especially in her dislike of his masculinity and her prudish distaste of the male genital. At one point he explained that he wanted to co-operate with his analysis but lacked trust in Klein, who he felt reproached him endlessly for his 'bad sexuality'. In his view, she was driving him mad and then planning to have him locked up.

The Dream of His Mother and the Bull as a Combined Parental Object

The hostility between Mr B's parents was expressed in a dream in which he saw a bull in a farmyard lying between himself and his mother. The bull looked uncanny and dangerous not fully alive, but also not quite dead. Mr B managed to escape, but felt that he was leaving his mother behind in danger. Klein suggests that his dream represents his phantasy of what happened between his parents, namely that theirs was a dangerous intercourse which threatened to kill his mother. Later that evening he received news that his mother had died, but in the next session he delayed mentioning this and instead expressed his fear that his treatment was going to lead to his death. Klein interpreted that his mother had become mixed up with the attacking bull father – half-dead himself – and had become uncanny and dangerous. She added that she had come to stand for this combined parent-figure, and that the increase of hatred against her and his mother was a defence against his sorrow and despair about his mother's death.

> I myself and the treatment were at the moment standing for this combined parent-figure. I pointed out that the recent increase of hatred against his mother was a defence against his sorrow and despair about her approaching death. I referred to his aggressive phantasies by which, in his mind, he had changed his father into a dangerous bull which would destroy his mother; hence his feeling of responsibility and guilt about this impending disaster. (Klein, 1940, p. 148)

It was typical of Klein that she also recognised her patient's loving side, which accounted for his feelings of sorrow for the damage that his violence had produced. After the bull dream, he was surprised that he had an association to some blackbirds, birds which he liked, but which had woken him that morning. Klein interpreted that they stood for his parents, whose intercourse disturbed him in the night but whom he also loved.

After his mother's funeral, Mr B's paranoia returned and he complained that he had to 'fight for his life' in his analysis. He had more violent dreams and declared that 'death was claiming him'. In one dream an out-of-control bus was crashing into a shed, and two people came from behind him and began opening the roof of the shed and looking into it. He could see no point in this activity, even though they seemed to think it would help him. Klein interpreted that the two people represented herself and the patient studying him together, and she understood that he found this a persecution rather than a help. She linked his reluctance to face his recent loss of his mother with his inability to face early infantile losses, which had produced the depression which he had been warding off all his life.

The revival of these early depressive feelings made the current mourning more difficult, but when the losses had been to some extent worked through, he was able to make significant steps towards feeling sorrow and guilt, and not just rage, towards his parents and towards Klein.

The patient's unconscious phantasy of his parents' relationship was one of mutual hostility. He seemed to believe that his mother's contempt of his father and of his sexuality led his father to feel humiliated and hostile, but also that their mutual hostility bound them in a relationship that excluded him and led in turn to his own humiliation. The evidence for this view arose from images such as those of the dangerous bull in the farmyard dream and of the bus out of control crashing into the shed and of the couple taking off the roof of the shed to look into it. However, if we turn to the *Lectures* (Steiner, 2017) and the *Narrative* (English, 2023), additional material becomes available that helps to clarify the patient's transference struggles with Klein and provides further information on his early childhood, which also helps us to understand what her idea of a combined parental couple meant.

Material from the Archives

A great deal more is known about Mr B from the *Lectures on Technique* (Steiner, 2017) and from Klein's clinical notes, published as *The Narrative of an Adult Analysis* (English, 2023). There is information about Mr B's background and some further details of the sessions around his mother's death in which the dream of the bull leads to the discussion of the combined object. Most significant, however, is the account of Mr B's meeting a child patient of Klein's, to which he responded with great distress and hostility. Klein was able to connect the sense of betrayal that he felt to a similar reaction from his childhood when his sister was born.

Background

When he began his analysis in 1934, Mr B was in his late twenties, with a wife and three children. Christine English (2023) discovered that this was about a month after the death of Klein's son Hans, and it is difficult to avoid the speculation that working with Mr B reminded her of the loss of Hans and created a link in her mind between the two people discussed in her paper on mourning. Mr B's mother died two years after his analysis began, and the treatment continued – with interruptions – for 12 years, until 1946. During the war, the patient served in the army, and was able to attend some sessions when he was on leave.

Humiliation Provoking Hostility

We saw how important feelings of humiliation were in the case of Mrs A, where they provoked hostility and a wish to triumph over her brother and mother, and then over her son. Similar feelings arose in Mr B's belief that his mother had looked down on his father and that the hostility that made him so dangerous arose from feelings that she had humiliated his father, particularly with her dislike of his sexuality. Despite their hostility to each other, his parents were also experienced as combining to exclude and humiliate him. In the archives, the cruelty of this combined object was illustrated in the way that when he misbehaved, his mother would hand him over to his father to be punished. His father would react brutally and smack him in the face, after which his mother would feel sorry but would repeat the pattern.

In his analysis, the patient tended to repeat the same kinds of complaints, especially that Klein emphasised the destructive side of his masculinity and did not sufficiently value his love and his wish to make reparation. These feelings emerged with great clarity when Mr B became enraged when he bumped into another of Klein's patients, a boy of about ten whose session she had had to move.

Meeting Another of Klein's Patients

The encounter with another of Klein's patients and its aftermath is described in the *Lectures on Technique*, and in greater detail in the *Narrative* (English, 2023, pp. 16–19). Meeting the child drastically disturbed Mr B's equilibrium and ushered in a long period of negativity in the analysis, which both patient and analyst found difficult. These sessions did, however, yield important information about the source of his hostility, which both Klein and the patient were able to link with the birth of Mr B's sister when he was five years old.

Klein had been obliged to change the session time of one of her child patients, which meant that Mr B met the boy leaving as he arrived. He overheard Klein talking to the boy as she escorted him out and he also heard the boy talking about him. His response was dramatic, and he furiously accused Klein of going back on her promise to preserve his session. At first, he tried to accept the situation and be reasonable, but he could not maintain this stance and his rage emerged with enormous vehemence. He would be silent only to burst out with accusations about how Klein had disappointed him and let him down. He repeatedly decided to stop his analysis but came every day, and before each session he struggled with his decision to break off. These struggles frequently made him very late, and he sometimes came only for a few minutes and stood by the door or sat at the far end of the couch.

Klein clearly found these sessions difficult; she tried to express her sympathy but also defended herself. She explained to him that she understood the hurt which had arisen from of the presence of the other patient, but pointed out that she had not actually altered his hour. To this Mr B replied that she had actually kept him waiting that day; Klein acknowledged that this happened to be true, but pointed out that it had been only by one minute! She then offered to change his time to start ten minutes later to avoid meeting the boy, but he refused, saying it would then not be his own hour anymore. When he was very late she would sometimes go over time by ten minutes, which he accepted but felt guilty about. She was able to convey that she understood that he could not help being late since there was too much anxiety connected with meeting the child. However, she also interpreted that the anxiety was less to do with his disappointment and more connected with the aggression that he felt towards the child and towards her. He seemed relieved when she said that in the current atmosphere, they would just have to be patient and do as much work as they could at the time.

In this period Mr B was depressed and angry, and spoke, for example, of feeling there was 'disaster all around him' and that he had '"fallen into a well of burning pitch"'. He also quoted a line from Coleridge: 'If we fall out with those we love/it works like poison on the brain'. In fact, this was a misquote, but it eloquently conveyed the distress he felt. Klein describes how, in this period, Mr B thought that everything about the analysis had become bad and everything that she had ever interpreted was wrong; he felt hopeless and simply wanted to break off his treatment. At one point he declared, 'you will not be able to do anything because my army is ready, and I am fully on its side' (English, 2023, p. 18). Nevertheless, there were moments of contact, and both Klein and Mr B himself recognised that the encounter with the other patient had reactivated his reaction to the arrival of the sister.

The Birth of the Patient's Sister

Mr B describes his sister's birth as a shattering experience of which he had no warning. At the time of his own birth, a nanny had been hired who became his beloved companion and shared his bedroom. Then at the age of five, something 'absolutely monstrous' took place. He had had no idea that a child was expected, and woke up one day to hear that a baby had arrived. Although his nanny remained kind, he felt he lost her, as well as his place in the nursery, when he was moved to sleep with his older brother, and he felt that his life was never the same again.

Mr B was particularly hurt that he was not allowed to lift or bath the baby, as if he were viewed as dangerous and his mother did not trust his loving feelings towards the infant. In a similar way, he accused Klein of only offering to change his session time to avoid his meeting her child patient because she did not trust him to control his aggression.

At the age of eight he was sent as a boarder to a prep school, and he complained that his mother did not even come with him to the school to say goodbye. He felt he was being turned out of his home, just as he had been turned out of the nursery. Klein understood the revival of these painful feelings as in support of her idea of his parents as a combined figure. Just as his mother and father combined to punish him, he felt that they combined in their decision to have him banished from the nursery. He saw them as linked in a relationship that led to his exclusion and humiliation and provoked feelings of hostility and resentment.

The Loss of the Ideal and the Phantasy of the Combined Parental Object

In her paper on mourning, Klein identifies the chief factors that block mourning to be hostility and triumph, which are at least sometimes associated with the phantasy of the combined parental object. Using the material from the archives, we can expand on this description and try to connect the hostility to other factors in the patient's situation at that time and in the childhood experiences these evoked. This was most striking, in the case of Mr B, when his hostility erupted with great violence after he met Klein's child patient. Although we do not know precisely how these factors were related to the death of his mother because these notes were undated (English, 2023, p. 16), his hatred suggests a store of resentment that had built up towards Klein. His grievance was specifically provoked by the shattering of an ideal relationship, and his fury became extreme, as he accused Klein of betraying her promise to protect this ideal represented by his session. He seemed to feel that he had been expelled from the special position he held in Klein's mind; the experience evoked earlier ones from his childhood and specifically those surrounding the birth of his sister, when he felt he was unfairly expelled from his place in the nursery and expected to cope as an older child.

Confrontations Over Power

The furious response to Klein led to a confrontation over power when Mr B felt he had been unfairly pushed into an inferior position and that he was looked down upon by Klein, whom he believed saw him as mad and wanted to have him put in an asylum. He did what he could to reassert his rights and to reverse his humiliation by triumphing over her. His disappointment was with an idealised object which had failed to fulfil his phantasy of uniqueness, and this led to a feeling of catastrophic collapse. Reality had intruded and he had to face the loss of the position of infinite privilege which he assumed had been promised. The loss eventually had to be mourned if he was to emerge from his depression and face the future, but mourning the loss was obstructed by his preoccupation with his grievance at having been unfairly treated. It was the hostility, driven by his grievance, that bound him to the lost object and that had to be dealt with before mourning was able to proceed.

The Universal Experience of Disillusion

Sodré has suggested that losing the illusion of an ideal relationship is a universal experience that always causes humiliation.[2] There is a catastrophic fall from a merging position of identification with the ideal object, 'I'm the breast', to a feeling of forced submission to the unbearable reality of separateness, need, and dependence. With the collapse of the superiority of the idealised couple, the patient feels small and looked down upon, and can only deal with the unbearable situation by reversing it in a triumph in which the loss is denied and the humiliation inflicted on the other. The longing for love is then replaced by a longing for power, and the patient inhabits an up-and-down universe, in which strength fuelled by hatred is idealised and love is seen as weak and contemptible.

In the case of Mr B, the grievance, with its righteous indignation at the loss of the ideal, led to the hostility towards Klein, which reflected the grievances he held towards his mother and that had been revived by her death. It was these grievances that prevented his mother's death from being mourned; his development was blocked while the patient and his analyst became locked in a mutual hostility that ensured that his melancholic state continued.

The Withdrawal of Projections as Part of the Work of Mourning

While the case of Mr B serves to demonstrate the nature of the obstacles to mourning, that of Mrs A can allow us to examine what goes on as the work of mourning proceeds. The central issue of separating the self from the object is beautifully shown in the dream in which Mrs A allows her son to fall to his death while she pulls herself away towards life. It is this act of separation that requires the loss to be accepted and depends on an acceptance of the verdict of reality. The consequence of this acceptance is that libido is withdrawn from the object and made available to be invested in new relationships.

In his emphasis on the withdrawal of libido, Freud was using the language of drive theory, which we are now able to supplement with an object relations formulation of the process. This suggests that, in addition to the withdrawal of libido, it is elements of the self that have previously been projected into the object that are withdrawn, and that this is what establishes a separateness between self and object.

The Internalised Object in Melancholia as a 'Composite-Object'

In his discussion of the predisposition to melancholia, Freud proposed that the relationship between the self and the internal object of melancholia is

2 Personal communication, 2012.

essentially narcissistic. Later he would describe this as depending on an identification.

> Children like expressing an object-relation by an identification: 'I am the object.' 'Having' is the later of the two; after the loss of the object it relapses into 'being'. Example: the breast. 'The breast is a part of me, I am the breast.' Only later: 'I have it' – that is, 'I am not it'... (Freud, 1941, p. 299)

A more recent understanding of narcissistic object relations (Rosenfeld, 1983) shows them to be based on the mechanisms of splitting and projection that lead parts of the self to be disowned and attributed to the object, and parts of the object being felt to belong to the self. Through projective identification, self and object are intermingled, leading to what might be aptly termed a 'composite-object'. We can then see that the act of separating self from object involves the withdrawal of parts of the self that have been imbedded in the object and returning them to the self. The verdict of reality can then also be seen to involve a judgement of what belongs to self and what belongs to the object, and leads to reassignments in which the self is enriched by gaining the previously disowned elements and the object is viewed more realistically and less distorted by projections.

Freud had been puzzled as to why the command of reality should be so extraordinarily painful that the withdrawal has to be done piecemeal (1917b, p. 245), and it often seems that the actual process of separating self from object is felt like a painful tearing apart. The pain was also evident in the case of Mrs A's dream, in which she had to watch her son fall to his death as she separated from him.

The Turning Point of Mourning

In these models drive theory remains useful, especially if we use the French *investissement* to describe the cathexis of libido (Laplanche and Pontalis, 1967). We can see that a critical change in the direction of the investment takes place at what can be considered to be a turning point in mourning (Steiner, 2023c). This point is associated with several interrelated changes. The acceptance of loss, the redirection of libido, and the return of projections are closely related, as is another development, namely that of a capacity for symbolic function. Until this turning point, the composite-object is experienced concretely, often as an uncomfortable weight in the chest or abdomen. The demands for reparation and revenge are also concrete and become burdensome and heavy. We still do not understand the full nature of the change to symbolism, nor why it should be related to the turning point of mourning, but it is clear that it has enormous consequences for the patient. When the concrete internalised lost object is replaced by its symbolic counterpart, the patient feels freed up from the burdensome duties towards the lost object and allowed to participate in the world of the imagination, to make use of dreams and fantasies, and, in particular, to make symbolic reparation rather than concrete repair. Quite how symbolism develops remains to a degree obscure, but it does seem that it is associated with the giving up of the lost object as a concrete possession. Segal (1957) argued that when projections are removed, the self and the object become more separate, and in turn the symbol and the thing symbolised can also become more separate. Subjectively, the change involves a shift from the hostility of grievance to the sorrow of loss, which is often associated with a breakdown into tears. The relief that is brought by tears was described by Klein in the cases of both Mrs A and Mr B.

The Softening of Grievance as Hostility Turns to Sorrow

Klein mentions that in the early stages, Mrs A rarely wept, and when she did it brought no relief. Later, however, she cried abundantly and felt the relief that comes with tears. Mr B failed to weep at the time of his mother's death, but at a later time, he broke down in tears and felt relief as he wept copiously. The weeping was brought on by a discussion of the way that children, particularly boys, are discouraged from crying and always expected to be cheerful, which suggested that he felt he ought to keep his emotions hidden, where they were locked away and in danger of fuelling a resentment. Now, as he could weep and felt free to liberate his tears, he went on crying hard for some time and spoke of 'the relief which one gets from tears' (English, 2023, p. 100).

When mourning is blocked by grievance, the subject often feels he is obliged to harden his heart against his oppressors. This was expressed by Mr B when he told Klein that he felt sympathy for the Pharaoh, who hardened his heart against Moses as God inflicted more and more plagues on him. At the time he had complained that Klein was being omniscient, knowing everything, like God, and making him feel attacked and humiliated.

The need to be tough and hard is poignantly put by King Lear when he claims, in his grievance against his daughters, that he would rather his heart break into fragments than soften.

> You think I'll weep;
> No, I'll not weep. – [Storm and tempest]
> I have full cause of weeping; but this heart
> Shall break into a hundred thousand flaws,
> Or ere I'll weep. – O fool, I shall go mad!
> (*King Lear*, 2.4, 471–474)[3]

3 In Bate and Rasmussen's edition this is Act 2, Scene 2. The line numbers are taken from that edition: J. Bate and E. Rasmussen (eds.) (2007), *William Shakespeare: Complete Works* (Houndmills: Macmillan).

I think, like Lear, that Mr B feared the conflict would drive him mad and that he longed to be able to break down into tears. The depressed patient often expresses the wish to be able to soften and relent, as does Hamlet, who expresses this longing as he says

> O that this too too solid flesh would melt,
> Thaw, and resolve itself into a dew!
> (*Hamlet*, 1.2, 129–130)

Like Lear he cannot do so, however, until the end of the play, because his resentment against his mother and her premature marriage is too strong.

> That it should come to this!
> But two months dead: nay, not so much, not two:
> (1.2, 137–138)

Weeping seems to mark the shift from grievance to grief and indicates that the turning point of mourning is near, but it is commonly resisted because it is felt to be weak and feminine and to undermine the masculine values of courage, loyalty, and honour that bind the mourner to the lost object. Indeed, the capacity to shift from the fortress mentality that characterises grievance and risk the vulnerability of softening may require an internal strength in order to be able to tolerate the embarrassment associated with weeping.

What Determines the Change from Grievance to Sorrow

Of course, the question of what facilitates a shift from the up-and-down world of hostility and triumph to enable mourning to proceed remains largely unanswered. It is the question that every analyst who is working with a patient who is trapped in cycles of grievance and revenge longs to answer. The shift seems related to the possibility of a softening in the warlike attitude that has developed, and the answer remains obscure. Sodré has suggested that the humiliation associated with the loss of the ideal is the experience that provokes the wish for revenge, and that sometimes the analyst can support the patient to endure the humiliation rather than to reverse it by inflicting it on the object.[4] She has argued that when the dethronement from the ideal leads to the fall into a position of humiliating inferiority, the mother can sometimes save the day if she can rescue the baby from the abyss by bending down to pick it up and return it to the family. Lowering herself to the level of the baby makes her seem less superior, and her empathic stance suggests that she knows from her own experience how painful disillusion can be. However the child inevitably wants to restore the

4 Personal communication, 2012.

phantasy of superiority for itself, and it is sometimes difficult to persuade it that there is enough love for it to be shared with the father and siblings. Nevertheless, a compassionate attitude, combined with a respect for the reality of family rivalries and tensions, is a useful model for the analyst even though it commonly fails to achieve the desired end.

Another idea that I put forward in Chapter 4, which looked at the 'Wrath of Achilles' as depicted in *The Iliad* (Steiner, 2025a), is that nothing can change until the grievance is externalised in all its violence, and revenge is enacted, to the point where the damage it has done is impossible to deny. Then perhaps the victory with its triumphant pleasures can give way to regret, sorrow, and the wish to make reparation. This idea, however, begs the question of how such a change can be achieved.

Our ignorance of how and why the changes at the turning point take place should not detract from the importance of observing them when they occur, and recognising that they may be times of acute sensitivity in the patient. We are helped if we remember Freud's observation that such changes are extremely painful, and become aware that part of the pain is associated with the shame of losing face that giving way involves. The moments of change can be impressive even if they are subsequently reversed and, as Freud warned us, need to be frequently repeated. This means that being with a patient who is gradually and painfully facing the suffering of loss can demand of the analyst both patience and devotion to their task, often represented by the stability of the analytic setting and the analytic attitude. Yet it is this quality that is often most appreciated, as it is associated with the analyst's ability to give up their own phantasies of omnipotent cure.

6 To Modify or to Defy the Super-Ego

Revisiting 'The Ego and the Id'[1]

Introduction

This chapter was included in a volume of *The International Journal of Psychoanalysis* commemorating the centenary of the publication of Freud's 'The Ego and the Id' (Freud, 1923). Klein admired 'The Ego and the Id', which laid the foundation for a structural theory of the mind, but she began to differ from Freud in interesting ways. They both saw defences against an unconscious sense of guilt to be of great importance, but Freud attributed these to repression while Klein saw them more in terms of splitting and projection. Indeed, the paranoid defence against guilt was one of her important formulations.

In accord with Strachey, Klein thought it was important to try to modify the severity of the super-ego, but she also admitted with Freud that it was often impossible to do so. In this chapter, I argue that in such cases the patient may have to accept the disappointment that the super-ego won't change and to find the strength to stand up to it. Here Britton's idea of emancipation of the ego from the dominance of the super-ego becomes critical (Britton, 2018).

I divide this paper into three parts. First, I discuss Freud's ideas about repression and the unconscious sense of guilt in order to compare them with Klein's view that we disown uncomfortable facts through a process of splitting and projection, leading to a paranoid defence against guilt. Second, I describe Klein's struggle to understand the origin and the severity of the primitive super-ego, which was so prominent in her child patients. She considered that an important aim of analysis was to moderate the severity of the super-ego in order to create a more humane inner world. Finally, I will elaborate on her view, as well as Freud's, that some of the primitive terrifying objects that lie buried deep in the unconscious are fixed and unmodifiable. I will use some ideas from Ron Britton to suggest that instead of trying to modify or get rid of these persecuting figures, it might be possible to stand up to them and to emancipate the ego from the tyranny of the super-ego.

1 Based on J. Steiner (2023b). A Kleinian Appreciation of the Ego and the Id (1923–2023), *The International Journal of Psychoanalysis*, 104: 1110–1120.

DOI: 10.4324/9781003726135-7

'The Ego and the Id' is one of Freud's most important works and is generally appreciated as a classic in which he establishes his structural theory of the mind. In the first two chapters, 'I. Consciousness and What Is Unconscious', and 'II. The Ego and the Id', Freud explains that he had come to reject the topographic model after realising that the distinction between consciousness and the unconscious was not as important as he had once thought. When considering the problem of the unconscious sense of guilt, he realised that the very agency that led to repression was itself unconscious, and this led him to replace the unconscious with a newly defined 'id', and the conscious with the 'ego', which was only partly conscious. Of course, the structural model represented a momentous advance but, for me, the originality of 'The Ego and the Id' lies in the description it gives of the super-ego and its relations with the ego. In fact, the paper should really have been named 'The Ego and the Super-Ego' rather than 'The Ego and the Id'.

In 'Chapter III. The Ego and the Super-Ego (Ego Ideal)', we hear how the super-ego arises in response to the loss of a sexual object and through its internalisation, introduces us to the idea of an internal world made up of objects in relationships.

> When it happens that a person has to give up a sexual object, there quite often ensues an alteration of his ego which can only be described as a setting up of the object inside the ego, as it occurs in melancholia; the exact nature of this substitution is as yet unknown to us. (Freud, 1923, p. 29)

Here, what is set up in the ego is the beginning of the super-ego. In 'Chapter IV. The Two Classes of Instincts', the destructiveness of the super-ego in its attacks on the ego is referred to as 'a pure culture of the death instinct', with a hint that it partly arises from the projection of the patient's sadism:

> Following our view of sadism, we should say that the destructive component had entrenched itself in the super-ego and turned against the ego. What is now holding sway in the super-ego is, as it were, a pure culture of the death instinct, and in fact it often enough succeeds in driving the ego into death, if the latter does not fend off its tyrant in time by the change round into mania.
>
> (Freud, 1923, 53)

In 'Chapter V. The Dependent Relationships of the Ego', the negative therapeutic reaction is described and associated with the need to deal with unconscious guilt, but Freud also puts forward the idea of an envious super-ego preventing pleasure and development.

All these findings led to a deeper understanding of the internal world and the objects it contained that profoundly influenced Klein and her followers. She deeply admired Freud's work, and I suspect that in her rivalry with Anna Freud she was disappointed that he did not give her own contribution similar attention. In fact, one of his few references to Klein was made in relation to the severity of the super-ego: 'Experience shows, however, that the severity of the super-ego which a child develops in no way corresponds to the severity of treatment which he has himself met with.' Freud's footnote adds: 'As has rightly been emphasized by Melanie Klein and by other English, writers' (Freud, 1930, p. 130 and footnote 1).

She freely acknowledged her indebtedness to Freud, particularly for the great discoveries of introjection, projection, and identification that she incorporated and developed in her own work:

> We owe to Freud and Abraham the great discovery that introjection and projection are of major significance both in severe mental disturbances and in normal mental life. I have here to forgo even the attempt to describe how in particular Freud was led from the study of manic-depressive illness to the discovery of introjection which underlies the super-ego. He also expounded the vital relation between super-ego and ego and the id. (Klein, 1959, p. 250)

Klein certainly saw the structural model of the mind as a major advance, and especially appreciated Freud's view that the super-ego was based on the internalisation of lost objects. For her, the internal world was structured by the way object relations were organised in unconscious phantasy (Segal, 2001), and she thought of the mind as structured by the internalisation of objects and their relationships.

The Paranoid Defence against Guilt and the Development of Grievance

I will begin by contrasting Freud's formulation, in which guilt becomes unconscious by being repressed, with that of Klein, in which guilt is split off and projected outwards.

In the first two chapters of 'The Ego and the Id', Freud struggled with the problem of unconscious guilt – how it was repressed and the nature of the moral force that led to the repression. For the most part Freud thought of the ego as unitary, distorted by pressure from the super-ego – rather like a rubber ball, deformed but not split. He did, however, write a paper called 'Splitting of the Ego in the Process of Defence' (1938b), which elaborated a theme developed in his paper on fetishism (Freud, 1927). There, he had described the recognition and simultaneous disavowal of an observation, such as the facts of sexual difference, and in 'An Outline of Psycho-analysis', he made a similar distinction, suggesting that

> ... what occurs in all these cases is a psychical split. Two psychical attitudes have been formed instead of a single one – one, the normal one, which takes account of reality, and another which under the influence of the instincts detaches the ego from reality. (1938a, p. 202)

For Freud, however, splitting was not yet connected with projection, although to my mind he came close to this idea when he described how the paranoia that can develop in melancholia could result from the investment of libido into the object. He could then argue that the paranoia can only be reduced if the libido can be withdrawn from the super-ego and returned to the ego:

> The cure, too, of such paranoic attacks would lie not so much in a resolution and correction of the delusional ideas as in a withdrawal from them of the cathexis which has been lent to them. The alternations between melancholia and mania, between a cruel suppression of the ego by the super-ego and a liberation of the ego after that pressure, suggests a shift of cathexis of this kind. (Freud, 1927, p. 165)

Freud seems to see the ego responding to pressure from the super-ego by the creation of a paranoid delusion, and subsequently the ego being liberated by the removal of the cathexis from the object. This seems to anticipate the formulation I will develop below, which uses the ideas of splitting and projection and suggests that a liberation of the ego is achieved through the withdrawal of the projections from the object and the returning of them to the self.

In Klein's theory, the ego is seen as constantly subject to splitting. Sometimes it is broken into fragments in a violent, chaotic way, and sometimes the splitting involves a more coherent process whereby a part of the ego is split off and projected. The former type of splitting, usually called pathological splitting or fragmentation, arises predominantly in psychotic or pre-psychotic states and results in an experience of the self as in bits; it is usually associated with massive anxiety, and often with depersonalisation (Rosenfeld, 1947). The anxiety of pathological splitting may be relieved if the fragments are projected into an object where they can be integrated and given meaning in a process described by Bion as 'containment' (1962).

Here, however, we are more concerned with the second type of splitting, also described in Klein's *Notes on Some Schizoid Mechanisms* (1946), in which part of the ego is split off and is attributed to the object through projection. This involves a split between good and bad elements of the self, in which usually it is the bad part that is projected and disowned. In this process the object is also split into a good part, with which an idealised relationship is created, and a bad one that offers only persecution. With everything bad split off, the good part of the ego can enjoy the idealised relationship, for example with the mother as the good object, thus creating what I think of as a Garden of Eden Illusion wherein the father and siblings are excluded (Steiner, 2018).

The split-off bad object does not disappear, however, but becomes internalised as a persecuting super-ego through which a moral universe of right and wrong is created. Freud vividly described how the self-reproaches of melancholia arise from an identification with these internalised bad objects, and showed that the underlying object relationship was between the self and the object in a state of mutual disappointment and grievance against each other. This leads to the humiliating self-abasement of the melancholic, which is commonly interspersed with periods of mania, creating an up-and-down world, in which either triumph or humiliation prevails.

While concepts such as splitting, projection, and projective identification can be viewed as original ideas developed by Klein, they were not only based on the work of Freud but were often anticipated by him. In 'The Ego and the Id', we are offered a detailed description of the history of the super-ego (using the basic findings from 'Mourning and Melancholia' (Freud, 1917b) as well as an outline of the mechanisms of identification and internalisation that lead to a model of an internal world in which objects interact in complex ways. When Freud said that the super-ego was the heir to the Oedipus complex, he established the idea of an internal world structured by the parents in a relationship with each other: 'The broad general outcome of the sexual phase dominated by the Oedipus complex may, therefore, be taken to be the forming of a precipitate in the ego, consisting of these two identifications in some way united with each other' (1923, p. 34).

Klein accepted Freud's structural model, although I don't think she assigned a huge importance to the id as a specific structure, instead seeing impulses and desires as arising within the ego:

> Freud's formulation of mental structure in terms of id, ego and super-ego has become the basis for all psycho-analytic thinking. He made it clear that these parts of the self are not sharply separated from one another and that the id is the foundation of all mental functioning. The ego develops out of the id, but Freud gave no consistent indication at which stage this happens; throughout life the ego reaches deep down into the id and is therefore under the constant influence of unconscious processes. (Klein, 1958, p. 84)

While she describes the ego as having developed out of the id, she mostly seems to use the id as a shorthand for that part of the ego from which wishes and desires emanate. She was developing an object relations theory, but wanted to leave room for drives. It is here that the idea of the ego as a body-ego seems most apposite. In this view, a part of the ego expressing unwanted wishes could be split off, projected, and identified with the object, a mechanism that was later to be called projective identification. For Klein, guilt did not simply disappear into the unconscious but became located in objects, and this process led to a relationship she referred to as the paranoid defence against guilt. In fact, it is said that she considered this idea to be her single most important discovery.[2]

2 I have not been able to corroborate this story.

Biographical Example of a Paranoid Defence against Guilt

As an example of the paranoid defence against guilt, I want to look at the situation of mutual grievance that develops between siblings vying for possession of their mother's love. The grievance follows an event which is deeply resented as unjust. One child feels themselves innocent and wronged while implicating the other as the cause of the trouble. The other, however, feels equally outraged, and a state of mutual grievance develops where each feels in the right and each insists that the guilt remains firmly attributed to the other. To the participants it is an all-or-nothing affair, while to an impartial observer the reality of what happened and who is responsible is more complex. However, passions are so high that no realistic examination of what actually took place can be envisaged.

Quarrels between brothers have been a feature in human history since the murder of Abel by Cain, and the rivalry that develops over possession of the mother's love is well illustrated by a striking instance reported in Richard Holmes' biography of Samuel Taylor Coleridge (2005):[3]

> In the autumn of 1779, when he was seven, a quarrel took place between Sam and Frank [his older brother] which throws much light on the psychology of the youngest son, and which Coleridge himself shrewdly presented as a formative event. ... It began ... in the kitchen of the Vicarage, in a dispute about food – and favouritism. Sam, typically demanding, had asked his mother to prepare him some special sliced cheese for toasting. Frank stole in, and minced it up 'to disappoint the favourite', and a violent fight ensued. Fifteen years later Coleridge still entered into the drama as he wrote.
>
>> I returned, saw the exploit, and in an agony of passion flew at Frank – he pretended to have been seriously hurt by my blow, flung himself on the ground, and there lay with outstretched limbs – I hung over him moaning & in a great fright – he leaped up, & with a horse-laugh gave me a severe blow in the face – I seized a knife, and was running at him, when my Mother came in and took me by the arm – I expected a flogging – & struggling from her I ran away, to a hill at the bottom of which the Otter flows – about one mile from Ottery. ...
>
> Sam fled ... to his old friend the river, ... and he remained there for the entire night ... He said his prayers, and thought *'at the same time* with inward & gloomy satisfaction, how miserable my Mother must be!' ...
>
> His mother, indeed, was 'almost distracted'. ... half the town had turned out to search for the missing child ... and 'no one went to bed'. At five in the morning Sam awoke, now frozen through, and too weak to move ... [His cries were by good luck heard by a neighbour, who carried him in his arms to his father]

3 This quarrel is also described in Chapter 4.

> 'I remember, & never shall forget, my father's face ... and the tears stealing down ... My Mother, as you may suppose, was outrageous with joy...'.
>
> Coleridge added that 'neither Philosophy or Religion' would allow him to forgive a local lady who suggested that he should have been whipped for this exploit. (Holmes, 2005, pp. 16–17)

We recognise that Sam's pride as well as his health was injured, and can imagine that after the fight his relationship with Frank was incompletely resolved, leaving behind a grievance and a wish for revenge. Nevertheless, we can imagine that unconscious guilt played a large part in Coleridge's personality and in both the mania and depression he suffered from throughout his life. Holmes tells us of further sources of guilt; some two years after the fight, Frank, at the age of 12, departed for a career in the Navy, and their father, on the night of his return from seeing him off, developed a fever and died. Then, to cap it all, as if by divine retribution, Frank committed suicide by shooting himself in a fever in India at the age of 22. It is, moreover, possible here to see a link to the terrible grievance that developed between Coleridge and Wordsworth, which was never resolved (Holmes, 2005).

In the passion of his rage, self-examination was impossible; Coleridge saw Frank as guilty of an unwarranted attack on his cheese and on the relationship with his mother that this represented, while no doubt Frank had his own version of the hurt that Coleridge inflicted on him through his favoured position with his mother. In the heat of the battle, however, one party is believed to be all good and the other all bad, and this continues to be the case when the wound is internalised as a grievance. Similar issues of pride may draw nations into wars, both hot and cold, in which the enemy is viewed as all bad.

Juliet Mitchell (2013, 2022) has described how with the birth of the next sibling the toddler feels ejected from the idealised relationship with the mother and feels thrown out of the family into the social world. Murderous feelings between siblings evolve into a state of war, which Mitchell suggests would lead to actual murder if it were not for what she calls the law of the mother, comparable to Lacan's law of the father. It is this law that enables the mother to intervene and prevent bloodshed, as we saw in the case of Coleridge. However, from the point of view of the child, the law of the mother represents a betrayal of her promise of idealised union in the Garden of Eden Illusion. Two objects of hatred then emerge: the brother with whom the war is waged, and the mother who betrayed him by making room for his brother in the family. As we saw, the withdrawal to his hiding place by the river was chiefly to hurt his beloved mother.

The grievance in response to wounded pride is very difficult to resolve, and is commonly nursed until it festers and traps the personality in a preoccupation with the need to project guilt. A persecuting super-ego is installed in the form of a reproachful internal object that demands restoration and revenge, and which leads to a mutually hostile relationship that cannot be relinquished and mourned. In thinking of this kind of grievance, it is important to remember that the super-ego is loved as well as feared. It is the betrayal by a loved and idealised object that creates the greatest wound, and there is always a hope that the feeling of being loved will be restored. Part of the dread is that the ego feels hated and persecuted by the super-ego, instead of loved (Freud, 1923, p. 288).

The longing to be loved is part of the poignancy of the grievance. The ideal object may be seen as the source of the persecution when it seems to be disappointed that we have not lived up to standards demanded by the ideal. It is this super-ego that Freud described so vividly in 'Mourning and Melancholia', and that later Klein was concerned to understand and, if possible, to modify.

Modifying the Severe Super-Ego: Can Projective Identification Be Reversed?

Klein was impressed with the extraordinary severity of the super-ego she observed in children, and considered that an important aim of analytic treatment was to reduce this severity. At first her argument was similar to that put forward by Strachey, who thought that the archaic super-ego could be modified if the patient experienced an interaction with a real, more benevolent analyst, which would enable the patient to recognise the contrast of this with the archaic persecuting internal figures:

> If all goes well, the patient's ego will become aware of the contrast between the aggressive character of his feelings and the real nature of the analyst, who does not behave like the patient's 'good' or 'bad' archaic objects. The patient, that is to say, will become aware of a distinction between his archaic phantasy object and the real external object. The interpretation has now become a mutative one, since it has produced a breach in the neurotic vicious circle. (Strachey, 1934, p. 143)

However, the original idea behind Klein's approach was the belief that the severity of the super-ego critically depended on what had been projected into it: 'For, when the objects are introjected, the attack launched upon them with all the weapons of sadism rouses the subject's dread of an analogous attack upon himself from the external and the internalized objects' (Klein, 1929, p. 438).

Later, when she developed her ideas on splitting, projection, and projective identification, a more detailed picture arose of the way objects are altered by being projected into. However, a reading of 'The Ego and the Id' makes it clear that Freud made the basic observations on which Klein's model was built, and the most important of these was that the super-ego arose from the internalisation of lost objects:

> When it happens that a person has to give up a sexual object, there quite often ensues an alteration of his ego which can only be described as a setting up of the object inside the ego, as it occurs in melancholia ....

> At any rate the process, especially in the early phases of development, is a very frequent one, and it makes it possible to suppose that the character of the ego is a precipitate of abandoned object-cathexes and that it contains the history of those object-choices. (Freud, 1923, p. 29)

Here Freud sometimes seems to be describing changes in the super-ego such as those seen in melancholia, while at other times it seems to be the case that it is the ego that undergoes alteration as a result of internalisation and identification. A critical factor is whether the lost objects were held onto and could not be fully mourned; indeed, it is these internalised objects that are identified with and form the character of the super-ego. Here we can turn to 'Mourning and Melancholia' to learn that a critical step in the work of mourning is for the subject to accept that the lost object is truly lost. A variety of mechanisms defend against this realisation, in particular the fact that the lost object is subjectively retained by means of the identification. When this happens, the external object is recognised as lost but is replaced by an internal object that functions as a super-ego. For mourning to proceed, the possession of this object must also be relinquished. Freud recognised that this second, internal relinquishment is painful and is vehemently resisted. In fact, it is so painful that it has to be done piecemeal, as '[e]ach single one of the memories and expectations in which the libido is bound to the object is brought up and hyper-cathected, and detachment of the libido is accomplished in respect of it' (Freud, 1917b, p. 245). Freud was still thinking in terms of libido, but the essence of his idea can be expressed in a more contemporary idiom if we think that the painful work of mourning consists in removing previously projected parts of the self and returning them to the ego (Steiner, 1996a). When successful, this process leads to a change in both the object and the self, the former becoming viewed in a more realistic light and the latter becoming enriched by regaining elements that had been disowned.

Moreover, another consequence of great significance is that the process of withdrawing projections is connected with the development of the capacity to symbolise. Quite how this happens remains to a degree obscure, but it does seem that, somehow, a symbolic representative of the formerly concrete internal object is able to evolve if possession of the lost object is given up. Segal (1957) argued that when projections are removed, the self and the object become more distinct, and this means that the symbol and the thing symbolised can also become more separate.

What is clear, however, is that grievance interferes with the process of mourning and leaves it incomplete. The grievance creates a link to the object and preserves its prominence in the mind of the patient. It is difficult to let go of the object, just as it is difficult to let go of the grievance, partly because the wrong associated with the grievance has not been put right. The mourner feels that there is unfinished business that must be concluded, usually through the triumph of revenge, before facing the loss becomes possible.

Here we must remember that the offending object is also the object that is loved, and whose love is yearned for. It is therefore often possible to detect a longing for a resolution, perhaps subjectively expressed as a wish to be free of the hard, frozen, concrete identification, and for it to be replaced with something softer and warmer. Hamlet seems to express this so well when he says

> O that this too too solid flesh would melt,
> Thaw, and resolve itself into a dew!
> (*Hamlet*, 1.2, 129–130)

He longs for something hard inside him to soften, but fears that the resulting flow of tears would be seen as feminine and thus make him feel too ashamed. Instead, he returns to the grievance and his wish to carry out his revenge (Steiner, 2023c). Perhaps it is in the flow of the tears that the object is finally relinquished and recognised as lost. Symbolic function can then evolve and, if the solid flesh can melt, the concrete object can be replaced by memories and phantasies created in the imagination. While much remains to be understood about this process, the consequences of symbolism are huge, especially in the area of reparation. Concrete objects such as those that form the melancholic super-ego demand concrete reparation, which inevitably fails. In a further twist that was brilliantly explored by Freud, an identification with the guilty object leads to the striking self-reproaches of the melancholic:

> While a melancholic can, like other people, show a greater or lesser degree of severity to himself in his healthy periods, during a melancholic attack his super-ego becomes over-severe, abuses the poor ego, humiliates it and ill-treats it, threatens it with the direst punishments, reproaches it for actions in the remotest past .... The super-ego applies the strictest moral standard to the helpless ego which is at its mercy; in general it represents the claims of morality, and we realize all at once that our moral sense of guilt is the expression of the tension between the ego and the super-ego. (Freud, 1933, pp. 60–61)

The Critical Importance of the Capacity to Make Reparation

The terrible dilemma facing the melancholic, and indeed to a degree all of us when we try to work through the process of mourning, was vividly described by Joan Riviere (1936) in her account of the pains of the depressive position. Weiss (2020) was so impressed with her account that he named the inability to fulfil the demand for concrete repair the 'Joan Riviere dilemma'. This involves a situation in which the individual feels unable to repair his damaged objects but is also unable to escape from their demands.

It is the concrete thinking that makes the reparation impossible, and both patient and analyst may become trapped in a concrete world dominated by despair. It is only when the possibility of concrete reparation based on magical and manic phantasies is abandoned that a shift towards symbolic reparation becomes possible. The difference was illustrated by Henri Rey[4] when describing a patient who complained of the impossibility of restoring her dead mother. Only gradually was she able to recognise that, by becoming a good mother to her own children, she was symbolically restoring a good mother inside herself. She was then able to imagine her mother's face with a smile when she saw her grandchild, replacing the more usual scowl. The reparation took place in her imagination rather than from the concrete actions that she had previously thought were necessary. When the work of mourning is brought to completion, the lost object is recognised as irreversibly lost and the subject can then negotiate what I think of as the turning point of mourning (Steiner, 2023c). This enables a move towards investing in the future rather than the past, whereas previously the severe super-ego demanded concrete reparation and prevented the acceptance of loss until this was achieved.

Standing up to the Primitive Super-Ego

Klein found abundant evidence in her child patients of primitive super-ego figures that seemed to reside permanently in the deep unconscious and were resistant to change. Moreover, she found that these 'extremely dangerous objects give rise, in early infancy, to conflict and anxiety within the ego; but under the stress of acute anxiety they, and other terrifying figures, are split off in a manner different from that by which the superego is formed and are relegated to the deeper layers of the unconscious' (Klein, 1958, pp. 86–87).

In a similar way, Bion found what he called an 'Ego-destructive super-ego', sometimes seeming to be motivated chiefly by envy:

> The super-ego figure on which strong envy has been projected becomes particularly persecutory and interferes with thought processes and with every productive activity, ultimately with creativeness. (Glover, 2009, p. 60)

These descriptions were anticipated by Freud, when he described an ego that feels hated and persecuted by a destructive, envious super-ego:

> The ego gives itself up because it feels hated and persecuted by the super-ego, instead of loved … [and so] … If we turn to melancholia … we should say that the destructive component had entrenched itself in the super-ego and turned against the ego. What is now holding sway in the super-ego is, as it were, a pure culture of the death instinct. (Freud, 1923, pp. 58, 53)

This kind of ego-destructive object is especially likely to come alive when we have alienated our good objects by rebelling against them and losing

4 Henri Rey, personal communication, 1966.

their approval and love, and this loss of approval is felt to be tantamount to a murder, because '[t]o the ego, living means the same as being loved – being loved by the super-ego' (Freud, 1923, p. 58).

Building on this work by Freud and Klein, Britton (2018) described how these extremely persecuting super-ego objects can dominate the ego and prevent any experience of pleasure or satisfaction. When this type of super-ego comes to dominate, there is nothing much that can be done, and it may present such a daunting prospect that both patient and analyst face feelings of despair in which all hope of relief are gone. However, out of this despair a new response of defiance can sometimes emerge, and instead of hoping for a more humane and benevolent super-ego the subject can decide to accept the super-ego as it is, try to live with it, and to stand up to it. Britton (2018) describes how this happened to Job in response to his persecution by God. He was obliged to submit outwardly, and was yet able to cultivate and maintain the right to protest internally against his persecution.

The Emancipation of the Ego from the Super-Ego

Here Britton points to one area of ego function that the super-ego tends to usurp and that can reasonably be reclaimed by the ego; namely the function of making reality judgements. In fact, Freud seems to agree, since, in a footnote of 'The Ego and the Id', he acknowledges that he wrongly attributed the function of judgement to the super-ego: 'I seem to have been mistaken in ascribing the function of "reality testing" to this super-ego – a point which needed correction' (Freud, 1923, p. 28 n2).

Britton suggests that these judgements include the realistic evaluation of the self – that is, deciding what is – while the super-ego passes moral judgements determining what should be:

> The separation of the ego from the superego can only be achieved by the ego using its most valuable function – that of observation and judgement – which it must turn on the superego. In other words, we must not simply be judged by our conscience; we must subject conscience to judgement. (Britton, 2018, p. 101)

It is this willingness to hold an opinion based on the right to make judgements that enables the ego to be emancipated even though the power of the super-ego remains unchallenged. Job submits, but privately gives free utterance to his complaint, something that Galileo was later to do in his outward compliance with religious authority.

Britton takes Job to be the ego and God to be the super-ego in this story, and understands this struggle to represent a crucial moment in analysis when the patient can question the authenticity of adverse judgements made by the analyst. This is particularly applicable to the problem of guilt, both conscious and unconscious. The super-ego may declare that to steal cheese from your brother is wrong, but the ego can demand to evaluate what actually did happen. What were the circumstances of the theft? Was his brother provoked? What amount of guilt is to be allocated to whom? Moreover, the ego reserves the right to make judgements of the super-ego. Did the mother betray the child by siding with his brother, and hence was the withdrawal into grievance justified or not?

By accepting the right to make judgements on what is happening, the ego is emancipated from the earlier dominance of the super-ego, and a reality principle can emerge alongside the morality principle espoused by the super-ego. On the other hand, the judgements inevitably demand a willingness to tolerate a realistic amount of guilt, proportionate to the wrongs done by each party.

The ability to stand up to the super-ego requires qualities such as strength, courage, and a respect for truth, which suggest the internalisation of strong supportive figures; this may involve a paradox because it is just these supportive figures that comprise the super-ego that is being challenged. Any new model will affect technique, and no matter how we try to observe analytic neutrality we can't help wanting the patient to stand up for himself. An important area of disappointment in analytic work arises when patients and supervisees try to follow what they see as an ideal model illustrated by an ideal analyst whom they do not dare to overthrow. It is not likely that much can be gained from directly encouraging the patient to rebel, because this only creates a double bind – e.g., 'Don't obey me!' But it may be possible to interpret a tendency to conform with a demanding super-ego which is never satisfied. This is probably a point that requires a paper of its own. Nevertheless, it does sometimes seem possible to internalise a father who is himself able to challenge authority and to establish the reality principle alongside the morality principle. A more objective reality recognises that both what is and what should be are important, and emphasises the relationship between them.

7 Romantic and Mature Love

'Tell me where is fancy bred'[1]

Introduction

The idealisation of romantic love is seen as a repetition of the early relationship between mother and baby, when, as two strangers, they see each other and fall in love. In his beautiful song 'Tell me where is fancy bred', from the casket scene of *The Merchant of Venice*, Shakespeare affirms that romantic love is linked to the gaze, but surprises us by introducing the theme of death in the midst of love. I argue that the recognition of loss and the work of mourning that results is what transforms romantic into mature love. This theme is developed to support Freud's contention, in his paper on the three caskets, that the lead casket represents death, which must be faced for love to become real and not superficial. With the acceptance of death, losses are faced and mourned, and love is more true when no longer idealised. It is argued that an ironic stance enables an acceptance of the pleasures of romance without believing them to be literally true.

In his short paper on the theme of the three caskets, Freud examines myths and folk tales to persuade the reader that in *The Merchant of Venice*, the choice between the three caskets is an example of the classical choice between three women. Portia, the beautiful and rich heiress, must be won by choosing the right one of three caskets of gold, silver, and lead. The right one is lead, and Freud argues this is because lead stands for death.

He finds evidence for this claim in numerous instances, including Cinderella, the Judgement of Paris, the Three Fates, and many other tales, of which his discussion of Lear and Cordelia is the most poignant. In the choice between his three daughters, Lear rejects the true one, whom Freud says stands for death because she 'loves and is silent'. He compares this to Bassanio's speech, in which he says of lead, 'Thy paleness moves me more than eloquence.' I wonder if Freud is not also moved by Cordelia's truthfulness. Her statement 'So young and yet so true' suggests that a true love accepts

1 Based on J. Steiner (2024), Differentiating Between Romantic and Mature Love: Revisiting the Three Caskets, *The International Journal of Psychoanalysis*, 105: 564–575.

DOI: 10.4324/9781003726135-8

the reality of death, perhaps here referring to Lear as an old man soon to die. Later, when Lear carries Cordelia's dead body onto the stage, Freud describes her as the death-goddess who, like the Valkyrie in German mythology, carries away the dead hero from the battlefield. Eternal wisdom, clothed in the primaeval myth, bids the old man 'renounce love, choose death and make friends with the necessity of dying' (1913a, p. 301).

In a similar manner, the choice of the right casket involves the acceptance of death as an inevitable feature of life, and the three caskets then represent

> – the woman who bears him, the woman who is his mate and the woman who destroys him. .... [And these] are the three forms taken by the figure of the mother in the course of a man's life – the mother herself, the beloved one who is chosen after her pattern, and lastly the Mother Earth who receives him once more. (Freud, 1913a, p. 301)

In this way, the three fundamental elements of life, birth, procreation, and death, are represented as aspects of a loved object, and the final inevitable outcome is death. I have tried to expand these observations, which seem to be profound and yet puzzling, since something as life-affirming as love is also associated with death. I have tried to link the need to accept the reality of death to the process of mourning through which romantic love is transformed into mature love. As a concrete reality, the ideal can then be relinquished and mourned but remains to be enjoyed in fantasy.

The Facts of Life

Psychoanalysts have viewed the three elements chosen by Freud as basic aspects of reality, poetically elaborated by Money-Kyrle as three fundamental facts of life. First, 'the recognition of the breast as a supremely good object', second, 'the recognition of the parents' intercourse as a supremely creative act', and third, 'the recognition of the inevitability of time and ultimately death' (1971, p. 103). The recognition of the breast as a supremely good object establishes the newborn infant's dependence on goodness that exists outside the self. It challenges the narcissistic illusion: 'The breast is a part of me, I am the breast' (Freud, 1941, p. 299). Money-Kyrle's second fact of life is really an extension of the first, because as soon as the mother is recognised to be a separate individual she is experienced as free to enter relationships with others. The prototype of these others is the father participating in an imagined or real sexual relationship, and the reality of the mother's freedom to love others is classically epitomised by the birth of a sibling. Sometimes even the freedom and independence of the mother is provocative when she is observed to be free to entertain her own thoughts.

Eventually, an awareness of time extends to the experience of waiting for ageing and death, which is so often 'forced on us, much against our will' (Money-Kyrle, 1971, p. 443). It begins with the awareness that good experiences do not go on for ever, and that the same is true of life itself. The passage of time seems to be difficult for all of us to accept, and even those who do not believe in an afterlife frequently search for utopias and deny the finality of death to gain comfort from illusions of immortality.

Because it brings home the reality of the passage of time and signifies that even things that seem perfect come to an end, death is the most fundamental obstacle for phantasies of eternal blissful love. If, on the other hand, the reality of time and death can be accepted, romantic love is able to develop and mature into a deeper love which can endure despite setbacks and ambivalences.

Death in *The Merchant of Venice*

Additional evidence from *The Merchant of Venice* supports Freud's contention that in the choice between the three caskets, lead stands for death and Bassanio's choice establishes death as a necessary part of life. Of course, the link between lead and death is confirmed by the properties of heaviness and dullness and by the fact that lead has long been used for coffins, but death also makes another unexpected appearance in the play – and perhaps its most striking – in the lovely song, 'Tell me where is fancy bred'. This song is performed while Bassanio is making his choice between the three caskets, and it leads us to ask what the role of death is, and why we should seek it in a love object. What makes Bassanio choose lead, and why did Portia's father make lead the correct choice?

The Choice between the Three Caskets

The episode of the three caskets takes place when the young soldier and scholar Bassanio, who has fallen in love with the rich and beautiful Portia, comes to woo her and to choose between the three caskets. He is poor and has had to borrow money from his friend Antonio, the merchant of the title of the play. Antonio in turn has had to borrow from Shylock on the surety of a pound of his flesh, and it is this debt, and the way it is demanded and then resolved, that forms the main theme of the play. The three caskets is a subsidiary theme, but one that sheds light on the characters of both Portia and Bassanio and the nature of the love between them.

Portia's father has devised a means of controlling and allegedly protecting his daughter by making her suitors choose between three caskets, one of gold, one of silver, and the third of lead. The lead casket contains her picture and leads to marriage, while making a wrong choice requires the suitor to leave immediately and to promise never to marry. The Prince of Morocco chooses gold, the Prince of Aragon silver, and Bassanio chooses lead, and wins Portia's hand.

Portia's independence of spirit is revealed early on when she complains to her maid that she has no choice in the outcome.

PORTIA:
But this reasoning is not in the fashion to choose me a husband. O me, the word 'choose!' I may neither choose who I would nor refuse who I dislike, so is the will of a living daughter curb'd by the will of a dead father. Is it not hard, Nerissa, that I cannot choose one, nor refuse none?
(*The Merchant of Venice*, 1.2, 14–18)[2]

Bassanio then arrives bearing gifts, declaring his love and his intention to take his chance with the casket. So far, his love is based only on glances they have exchanged, which emphasises the importance of gaze in romantic love. Here he describes his love to Antonio:

BASSANIO:
In Belmont is a lady richly left,
And she is fair, and, fairer than that word,
Of wondrous virtues. *Sometimes from her eyes*
I did receive fair speechless messages:
Her name is Portia [...]
(1.1, 163–167)

Bassanio is impressed with her beauty, to say nothing of her wealth, and these features of romantic love are based on glances and hearsay. He will be in for a shock when he is forced to recognise her wisdom and spirit. Portia's virtues attract numerous suitors, who come in quest of her Golden Fleece.

BASSANIO:
Nor is the wide world ignorant of her worth,
For the four winds blow in from every coast
Renowned suitors, and her sunny locks
Hang on her temples like a golden fleece,
Which makes her seat of Belmont Colchos' strand,
And many Jasons come in quest of her.
(1.1,169–174)

2 The quotations from *The Merchant of Venice* are from the Project Gutenberg eBook of *The Merchant of Venice*, by William Shakespeare. Publication Date: November 1998. Sonnet 138 is taken from the Project Gutenberg eBook of *The Sonnets*, by William Shakespeare. Publication Date: September 1997.

Portia herself seems in love, or ready to fall in love, on the basis of an earlier brief encounter with Bassanio, also described by her maid in terms of his looks.

> NERISSA:
> Do you not remember, lady, in your father's time, a
> Venetian, a scholar and a soldier, that came hither
> in company of the Marquis of Montferrat?
>
> PORTIA:
> Yes, yes, it was Bassanio, as I think, so was he call'd.
>
> NERISSA:
> True, madam. He, of all the men that ever my foolish
> eyes look'd upon, was the best deserving a fair lady.
>
> PORTIA:
> I remember him well, and I remember him worthy of
> thy praise.
>
> (1.2, 74–78)

At first, when Bassanio arrives, Portia pleads with him to delay his choice, and in doing so reveals her love for him. She is afraid that he might choose the wrong casket, and thinks of ways she might warn him, which she is forbidden to do.

> PORTIA [to BASSANIO]:
> I pray you, tarry. Pause a day or two
> Before you hazard, for in choosing wrong I lose your company.
> … I would detain you here some month or two
> Before you venture for me. I could teach you
> How to choose right, but I am then forsworn.
>
> (3.2, 1–11)

Portia even imagines music accompanying his failure:

> Then if he lose he makes a swan-like end,
> Fading in music. That the comparison
> May stand more proper, my eye shall be the stream
> And wat'ry death-bed for him.
>
> (3.2, 46–49)

The eyes again feature in the vision of her tears producing a watery deathbed for him. On the other hand, if he should win, the music would sound the birth of a new-crowned monarch.

> He may win,
> And what is music then? Then music is
> Even as the flourish when true subjects bow
> To a new-crowned monarch. Such it is

As are those dulcet sounds in break of day
That creep into the dreaming bridegroom's ear
And summon him to marriage.
(3.2, 49–55)

Away, then! I am lock'd in one of them.
If you do love me, you will find me out.
Nerissa and the rest, stand all aloof.
Let music sound while he doth make his choice.
(3.2, 42–45)

'Tell me where is fancy bred'

While Bassanio is pondering on his choice, the song 'Tell me where is fancy bred' is sung in the background, clearly within his hearing. The singer speaks for Portia and her household, who are all anxious that Bassanio should make the right choice.

SINGER:
Tell me where is fancy bred,
Or in the heart or in the head?
How begot, how nourishèd?
Reply, reply.

It is engend'red in the eyes,
With gazing fed, and fancy dies
In the cradle where it lies.

Let us all ring fancy's knell:
I'll begin it. – Ding, dong, bell.

ALL:
Ding, dong, bell.
(3.2, 65–74)

At first this lovely song seems to compare rational love coming from the head with emotional love from the heart, and the many words that rhyme with *lead, bred, head, nourished,* seem to be attempts to nudge Bassanio to the right choice. However, the singer replies that fancy is bred neither in the heart nor the head but in the eyes, which points to the fact that the eyes and the gaze play an important part in romantic love.

After asserting that fancy is 'engendered in the eyes/With gazing fed', the mood suddenly descends to announce fancy's death.

and fancy dies
In the cradle where it lies.

There is a precipitous fall from romantic love, however engendered, to death, which is unexpected and shocking. Here we are brought up against several questions which Shakespeare, in his usual manner, leaves open to many interpretations. Why does fancy suddenly die? Why in the cradle? And is there a pun intended when in the cradle fancy *lies*? And why indeed does the song end with an upturn of mood when the singer urges all to announce the death of fancy by ringing fancy's knell?

> Let us all ring fancy's knell:
> I'll begin it. – Ding, dong, bell.
>
> ALL:
> Ding, dong, bell.

Of course, we are free to speculate and imagine, even if no single meaning will exhaust the possibilities. It is difficult to avoid the idea that the sudden appearance of death represents the reality of the passage of time and hence the inevitable disillusion that follows romantic love. If this were to be so it could herald the acceptance of loss and hence the beginning of a move towards mature love. Perhaps the cradle refers to the gaze that has cradled the love, but it may also refer to the actual cradle and suggest that disillusion might happen early on in life when the baby feels put down and the idealised illusion of endless bliss with the mother is shattered.

Perhaps at birth the early relationship between the baby and the mother is of necessity romantic because they are, after all, strangers meeting for the first time and engaging each other through the gaze. The idealisation is interrupted when the mother's gaze no longer holds the baby and when her attention shifts to something else, for example to a husband or a sibling. The illusion held by the baby that he is his mother's partner in a romantic relationship collapses, and he falls into a humiliating realisation of his smallness and dependence. His shame is increased when he realises that the romance had been an illusion since all the time he had been supported at the breast by the mother's arms and held in her attention by her gaze. It may in fact be sufficient for the mother to turn to her own independent thoughts to make the baby feel dropped.

The Importance of Irony

This is perhaps one version of fancy dying in the cradle, but why does it lie? Here it is difficult to avoid a comparison with Sonnet 138:

> When my love swears that she is made of truth
> I do believe her though I know she lies,
> That she might think me some untutor'd youth,
> Unlearned in the world's false subtleties.
> Thus vainly thinking that she thinks me young,

Although she knows my days are past the best,
Simply I credit her false speaking tongue:
On both sides thus is simple truth suppress'd[.]

The poet's mistress pretends that he is young, which he knows is false but pretends to believe. They both know the truth but prefer the falsehoods, as the final couplet asserts.

Therefore I lie with her, and she with me,
And in our faults by lies we flatter'd be.

So, we might imagine the baby and the mother flatter each other with the illusion that their love is ideal and eternal. Here it makes a big difference if the illusion is recognised as such. The danger arises when the romantic couple, whether baby and mother or lovers entranced, take the illusion to be literally true and perfection is thought to have been realised and paradise achieved. It is only after disillusionment that they may continue to believe this even though they know it is a lie. Perhaps here, in the cradle, we find the earliest appearance of irony in our lives, which may then be established as a critical step on the path to mature love. It enables us to enjoy an illusion while remaining aware it is not quite real.

But why then is the singer so eager to toll fancy's knell, and for the others to join in: 'Ding, dong, bell'? As observers we can imagine that we feel excluded and grow tired of the endless bliss of the lovers' idealisation and that we long for something more real. Portia seems to move in this direction when she places obstacles in the way of the perfection of Bassanio's love. Perhaps she thinks he has had it too easy. He has borrowed money to woo her and put his friend at serious risk; he has guessed the right casket; and he is now a rich man with a beautiful wife. She herself has had the advantages of beauty and wealth, but she is also wise and aware that she must learn from experience. She is, moreover, not beyond playing a trick or two, as if she wants to push Bassanio towards a deeper, more truthful love, which can only be achieved if the idealisation is given up.

The Episode of the Rings

Portia's wisdom lies in self-knowledge, which makes her realise that she needs to develop and learn from experience. She sees herself as an

PORTIA [to Bassanio]:
... unlesson'd girl, unschool'd, unpractis'd;
Happy in this, she is not yet so old
But she may learn; happier than this,
She is not bred so dull but she can learn;
...

Happiest of all, is that her gentle spirit
Commits itself to yours to be directed,
As from her lord, her governor, her king.
(3.2, 162–168)

Portia is eager to learn, and her independence is suggested by the irony of the last two lines. Early in the play she was helpless in the face of her father's power to control her future, which she was unable to challenge. Now she has developed, perhaps helped by having to suffer her dismay with the unsuitable suitors, and makes clear that in her relationship with her husband she is no longer prepared to be passive and compliant. She will accept her husband as her governor and King, but also intends to teach him the painful lesson of disillusion that comes with loss. Through his marriage he has gained her wealth, her servants, and herself as his possessions, but Portia retains her independence. In a masterful ruse she gives Bassanio a ring, and threatens that its loss would mean that their love was ruined.

PORTIA:
This house, these servants, and this same myself
Are yours, – my lord's. I give them with this ring,
Which when you part from, lose, or give away,
Let it presage the ruin of your love,
And be my vantage to exclaim on you.
[gives BASSANIO a ring]
(3.2, 173–177)

Bassanio, in the manic triumph of his success, sees everything turned to joy, and makes light of the possibility of betrayal, asserting that only death would part him from the ring.

BASSANIO:
Where every something being blent together,
Turns to a wild of nothing, save of joy
Express'd and not express'd. But when this ring
Parts from this finger, then parts life from hence.
O, then be bold to say Bassanio's dead!
(3.2, 184–188)

The memorable judgement of 'the pound of flesh' is approached when news is brought of Antonio's misfortune. His ships are all wrecked, and the default on his bond means that Shylock can claim his pound of flesh. Portia displays her capacity for trickery once more when, disguised as a learned judge, she uses a legalistic quibble to demand that not a drop of blood be spilt when Shylock claims his bond. This condemns him and sets Antonio free, and again everything turns out well for Bassanio, whose guilt over placing Antonio in mortal danger is painlessly absolved. But here is where Portia introduces her ruse; in the form of a wise doctor, she demands Bassanio's ring as recompense for her judgement. Eventually the reluctant Bassanio is persuaded to hand it over, and has to face her anger on his return to Belmont. In fact, there has been a double wedding and a double betrayal, because Bassanio's friend Gratiano has fallen in love with Portia's maid Nerissa, and has also relinquished a ring she gave him with the same conditions. It is his scolding that Portia overhears:

> GRATIANO [to NERISSA]:
> By yonder moon I swear you do me wrong;
> In faith, I gave it to the judge's clerk.
> Would he were gelt that had it, for my part,
> Since you do take it, love, so much at heart.
>
> PORTIA:
> A quarrel, ho, already! what's the matter?
>
> GRATIANO:
> About a hoop of gold, a paltry ring
> That she did give me. ...
>
> NERISSA: ...
> Gave it a judge's clerk! No, God's my judge,
> The clerk will ne'er wear hair on's face that had it.
> (5.1, 152–168)

Nerissa accuses Gratiano of giving the ring to a woman; which, in fact, he did, since she was the judge's clerk. Portia plays the same conceit when she accuses Bassanio and swears that she will not sleep with him until she sees the ring.

> PORTIA:
> What ring gave you, my lord?
> Not that, I hope, wh ch you receiv'd of me.
>
> BASSANIO:
> If I could add a lie unto a fault,
> I would deny it, but you see my finger
> Hath not the ring upon it; it is gone.
>
> PORTIA:
> Even so void is your false heart of truth.
> By heaven, I will ne'er come in your bed
> Until I see the ring.
> (5.1, 195–202)

Bassanio pleads forgiveness and is confident in Portia's generosity once she is told of the circumstances.

BASSANIO:
Sweet Portia,
If you did know to whom I gave the ring,
If you did know for whom I gave the ring,
And would conceive for what I gave the ring,
And how unwillingly I left the ring,
When nought would be accepted but the ring,
You would abate the strength of your displeasure.
(5.1, 205–210)

Portia sticks to her ground.

PORTIA:
If you had known the virtue of the ring,
Or half her worthiness that gave the ring,
Or your own honour to contain the ring,
You would not then have parted with the ring.
(5.1, 211–214)

And then she carries the conceit further by accusing Bassanio of giving the ring to a woman, and in retaliation threatening to sleep with the good doctor herself.

PORTIA:
Let not that doctor e'er come near my house,
Since he hath got the jewel that I loved,
And that which you did swear to keep for me,
I will become as liberal as you,
I'll not deny him anything I have,
No, not my body, nor my husband's bed.
Know him I shall, I am well sure of it.
Lie not a night from home. Watch me like Argus, [the giant with 100 eyes]
If you do not, if I be left alone,
Now, by mine honour which is yet mine own,
I'll have that doctor for mine bedfellow.
(5.1, 235–245)

Portia continues to torment Bassanio, as if to drive the message home, while we the audience are confident that she will forgive him when she admits that she was the good doctor. We remember, after all, Portia's memorable speech:

The quality of mercy is not strain'd,
It droppeth as the gentle rain from heaven

> Upon the place beneath. It is twice blest,
> It blesseth him that gives and him that takes.
> (4.1, 184–187)

In due course all is revealed and all forgiven, as Portia explains her deception, which the two lovers failed to recognise.

> PORTIA:
> ... Here is a letter ...
> There you shall find that Portia was the doctor,
> Nerissa there, her clerk.
>
> BASSANIO:
> Were you the doctor, and I knew you not?
> ... Sweet doctor, you shall be my bedfellow.
> When I am absent, then lie with my wife.
> (5.1, 281–284, 295–300)

The Difference between Romantic and Mature Love

Faith is restored, but Bassanio has been through the ordeal of losing the love he so cherished and believed he was in possession of. To make the connection between loss of love and death, we can do no better than turn to Freud, who recognised that the loss of love of the object on whom we depend is treated as equivalent to its death.

> In melancholia, the occasions which give rise to the illness extend for the most part beyond the clear case of a loss by death, and include all those situations of being slighted, neglected or disappointed, which can import opposed feelings of love and hate into the relationship or reinforce an already existing ambivalence ... (Freud, 1917b, p. 251)
>
> But the free libido ... served to establish an *identification* of the ego with the abandoned object. Thus the shadow of the object fell upon the ego, and the latter could henceforth be judged by a special agency, as though it were an object, the forsaken object. ... the object-choice has been effected on a narcissistic basis, so that the object-cathexis, when obstacles come in its way, can regress to narcissism. (Freud, 1917b, p. 249)

Romantic love, so evidently narcissistic, is shattered when Bassanio is led to believe that he has lost Portia by losing the ring. A shadow has fallen over his ego, and he feels judged and condemned. When properly confronted, such a loss of love heralds the onset of the depressive position. To quote Klein,

> Here we see one of the situations which I have described as being fundamental for 'the loss of the loved object', the situation, namely, when

> the ego becomes fully identified with its good, internalized objects, and at the same time becomes aware of its own incapacity to protect and preserve them against the internalized, persecuting objects and the id. (Klein, 1935, p. 148)

Bassanio pleads for forgiveness, and as he faces the loss of Portia's love for the first time, he realises that it is unlikely to be the last. He has, after all, to contend with a wife who has given him all but has retained her independence of thought. Initially she was like lead, dumb and dull in her need to submit to her father's way of choosing a husband for her, but she has gradually come to enjoy a liveliness of spirit which can ensure her freedom of thought. Perhaps a young mother has initially to comply with the tyrannical demands of her infant, but is able to evolve into an independent person with her own mind. It is such independence that can be the trigger to the collapse of the idealisation of romantic love and the fall into depression and despair. It is through such painful contact with the separate existence of the other person that romantic love changes into mature love.

Perhaps all love begins as a romance between a couple attracted to each other at first sight, using only brief superficial observation supplemented by flights of imagination. Commonly romantic love manages to survive adverse events, but at other times it is setbacks, particularly the slights and disappointments that herald ambivalence, that are required for mature love to develop. Sometimes, indeed, a more pathological version of narcissistic object-choice can have serious consequences. Sodré (2013) has vividly described how some people become addicted to romantic daydreams which they try to realise without concern for reality. She shows how such phantasies can be tragically enacted and fail to mature into a realistic love. There are also psychotic versions of romantic love in which a delusional belief may fuel excitement and may turn into paranoia when the phantasy is not confirmed. In the transference, such phantasies may give rise to a variety of erotomania, in which a conviction develops that the analyst is in love with the patient.

Even the phrase 'fall in love' suggests a lack of volition, as if we are tripped and fall headlong into the object. By contrast, 'loving' is a transitive verb that indicates that love emanates from the self to reach the object that it apprehends and, despite its shortcomings, loves. Romantic love is idealised, often associated with endless bliss, in which time, loss, and death play no part. This is the nature of love in the Garden of Eden, which can be thought to represent the illusionary early perfection of love between the infant and the mother. Two strangers meet and fall in love by creating an illusion of the other and by projecting an image of what each desires. Ambivalence is avoided through splitting and projection until, in normal circumstances, reality breaks through and the couple is obliged to face a bitter disillusionment, in which the loss of the ideal is mourned before they can begin to properly understand each other and love each other.

If the reality can be accepted mature love evolves, and ambivalence, with its admixture of aggression, gives rise to guilt. The consequences are movingly described by Klein in her *Lectures on Technique*.

> I hold the view that feelings of sorrow, guilt and anxiety are experienced by the infant when he comes to realize to a certain extent, that his loved object is the same as the one he hates and has attacked and is going on attacking in his uncontrollable sadism and greed, and that sorrow, guilt and anxiety are part and parcel of the complex relation to objects which we call love. It is from these conflicts that the drive to reparation springs, which is not only a powerful motive for sublimations, but also is inherent in feelings of love, which it influences both in quality and quantity. (Klein, 1936, p. 37)

Mature love depends on the capacity to tolerate guilt and to use it to fuel the wish to make reparation to the loved one we have hurt and damaged.

Nevertheless, romantic love, with its basis in idealisation, plays a huge role in literature, music, art, and of course in real life, where it not only provides an escape from the ugliness and pain of the real world but liberates creative endeavours that lead to works of real beauty and significance. It should not be thought that when mature love has evolved that there is no place for romance. What changes, however, is that we recognise more and more that romance resides in the world of phantasy, illusion, and imagination, and in as much as we love maturely, we know that the ideal is not realisable in reality. At the same time, we become aware that it is the experience of loss and its working though by mourning that leads to an appreciation of the true value of the object. Perhaps we could adapt Tennyson's famous couplet and suggest that

> *Unless* one has loved and lost
> One has not truly loved at all.[3]

The choice of the lead casket with its association with death may thus make room for 'sorrow, guilt and anxiety' as 'part and parcel of the complex relation to objects which we call love', and support Freud's intuition that death plays a significant role in the choice of a loved one. We continue to enjoy the pleasures of romantic love, which we see as both true and false; we continue to believe it though we know it lies.

3 'Tis better to have loved and lost

Than never to have loved at all.
(*In Memoriam A. H. H.*,27.15–16)

8 Chaos, Freedom, and Order in the Analytic Setting[1]

Introduction

In this chapter I will examine the role of freedom in the analytic setting, where it commonly needs to be protected from excessive chaos on the one hand and excessive order on the other. The topic is highly relevant to our practice, not only because of the pressing issue of freedom in society but because of the importance of freedom of thought in the minds of our patients, which psychoanalysis values and attempts to liberate.

When anxiety is high, the analyst is pressured to give priority to safety, which the analyst attempts to provide through the regularity and structure of the analytic setting. This setting creates order by establishing a boundary within which the patient is safe and free to express themselves and to develop their own thinking. Sometimes, however, especially when the patient demands urgent relief, the authority of the analyst can become excessively controlling and rigid. The analyst may cope with their own difficulties by splitting and projection, and transform the boundary of the setting into a solid shield or wall to keep hostility and chaos at bay. The patient may welcome the safety that such containment provides, but the analytic function then comes to be experienced as an external shell or carapace, which relieves anxiety at the expense of freedom.

When they become stronger, the patient may resent the confinement provided by the rigidity of the shell and feel the protection to be so excessive and condescending that they seek to break free. To find the strength to rebel the patient turns to an external source of support, which is then internalised as a backbone or spinal column. I think of the containing function as maternal and, when under stress, in danger of becoming excessively controlling. The support to rebel and make a bid for freedom then requires a complementary paternal influence, which can also be a danger if it takes the form of phallic superiority, sometimes attacking the boundaries and reintroducing chaos

1 The chapter is based on a paper given to the Hungarian Psychoanalytical Society in October 2025. I am grateful to the organisers for the title of the conference, which also became the title of this chapter.

DOI: 10.4324/9781003726135-9

and sometimes imposing excessive order based on omnipotence. A balance between safety and freedom is required in which paternal and maternal influence moderate each other, and this depends on a balanced relationship between them.

I will turn to Freud, Klein, and others to explore this theme, including the description in *Paradise Lost* in which Milton shows how God circumscribed an area of chaos and in this way attempted to protect Eden's perfection when he created the world. I will also give two clinical examples, one of excessive chaos and one of excessive order, which I hope will show how internal conflicts become projected onto the transference relationship where the battle for freedom is worked through.

The Dangers of Omnipotence: Being Master of One's Mind

Chaotic thoughts can lead to the fear of loss of control of one's mind, a frightening experience which we usually associate with serious mental illness and breakdown. However, if we listen to Freud, perhaps taking him a bit literally, we are never truly in control of our own minds, and the illusion that we are masters there is based on omnipotent phantasy.

When he described just how difficult it is to be in control, Freud expressed his sympathy for the poor ego, which is obliged to struggle with three masters.

> The poor ego … serves three severe masters and does what it can to bring their claims and demands into harmony with one another. These claims are always divergent and often seem incompatible. No wonder that the ego so often fails in its task. Its three tyrannical masters are the external world, the super-ego and the id.
>
> …
>
> Thus the ego, driven by the id, confined by the super-ego, repulsed by reality, struggles to master its economic task … and we can understand how it is that so often we cannot suppress a cry: 'Life is not easy!' If the ego is obliged to admit its weakness, it breaks out in anxiety – realistic anxiety regarding the external world, moral anxiety regarding the super-ego and neurotic anxiety regarding the strength of the passions in the id. (1933, pp. 77–78)

Earlier Freud argued that it was the discoveries of psychoanalysis that had made us aware of our failure to control our minds, first because we cannot wholly tame our instincts and second because our mental processes are themselves unconscious. These two discoveries led to a shattering of the illusion that we are in control.

> … [They] amount to a statement that *the ego is not master in its own house*. Together they represent the third blow to man's self-love, what I may call the *psychological* one. (1917a, p. 143)

All three of these blows shatter narcissistic illusions. The first is the belief that the earth is the centre of the universe, disproved by Copernicus, and the second the idea that man has a special place in nature, disproved by Darwin. The final blow to the illusion of authority in man's own mind, which Freud thought was the most personally wounding, is the psychological blow that makes the ideal of mental mastery a hopeless dream.

Using the words 'master in his own house' suggests the *pater familias*, who since Roman times had had undisputed power to control his wife, children, and servants; Freud implied that we all have a secret longing to have this kind of mastery. This is particularly so when we feel small and helpless and get relief from phantasies of omnipotence. Mastery is sometimes felt to be necessary in the search for both safety and freedom, and comes into conflict with the demands of reality.

The Dread of Chaos and the Demand for Relief

Chaos disrupts trains of thought, creating fragmented thinking and confusion and leading to anxiety and fear of breakdown. In these situations, the discomfort may be extreme and lead to an urgent demand for relief in the form of containment and structure. In desperation, the patient may turn to any source of order, no matter how delusional. Chaos commonly arises when a containing structure has collapsed, for example when war or family disruptions expel the child from safety into chaos. Sometimes it is the breakdown of splitting that has led to a confusional state, while at others it is unrestrained impulses emanating from the id that create the chaos. In all these situations the urgency means that omnipotent solutions may be turned to at the expense of freedom, commonly in the form of an authoritarian system, which is internalised as an authoritarian super-ego. This means that a swing from excessive chaos may result in the establishment of excessive order. The severity of the super-ego may arise from the need to create an impregnable structure to keep disorder from intruding, and give rise to a fortress mentality.

The Controlling Super-Ego of Melancholia

Freud's descriptions of the internal world of the melancholic helps us to understand how a powerful super-ego becomes established as an internal entity exacting obedience and making concrete demands for reparation and revenge. The severity is increased through the projection onto it of the infant's own demands, as split-off parts of the self are projected and identified with the object. This deployment of projective identification gives rise to what I have called a *composite-object*, in which self and object are intermingled and not experienced as separate. Composite-objects prevent the development of symbolic function, and it seems to be the failure to separate which gives rise to concrete thinking (Segal, 1957). While the change from concrete to symbolic remains incompletely understood, it has important consequences. The concrete demands of the super-ego, for example, seem impossible to fulfil, and the burden is relieved if it can be expressed symbolically in dreams and phantasies.

When the super-ego becomes excessively controlling, it is natural to try to lessen its severity, and most analysts, including Klein (1940), follow Strachey (1934) and attempt to moderate its rigidity by analysing the conflict in the transference. It is, however, common to find that elements of the super-ego are resistant to change, and both Freud and Klein described monstrous objects in the deep unconscious that defy therapeutic efforts. If freedom of thought is to be recovered in these cases, it may be necessary to accept the severity of the super-ego and find the courage to stand up for oneself against it. It is here that a paternal support internalised as a backbone becomes important, and the weak ego whose self-confidence has collapsed under super-ego scrutiny needs to find a way of asserting itself (Freud, 1917a). Britton speaks of the need to emancipate the ego from the dominance of the super-ego (2018).

The Pleasures and Dangers of Omnipotence

Omnipotence confers advantages, especially if a weak ego is unable either to organise chaos or to rebel against order without it. In the short term it may be useful and even necessary but, in due course, its dangers must be recognised so that reality can prevail.

Another important function of omnipotent order is to enable splitting and strengthen the forces of good in the struggle against evil. Indeed, it is possible that a fourth fact of life that we could add to the three postulated by Money-Kyrle (1971) is the existence of evil – in others, but also within ourselves.[2] This is perhaps a corollary of Freud's death instinct and Klein's postulate of the universality of envy. The function of an omnipotent leader is to ensure order by splitting off evil and attributing it to real or potential enemies. Thus, Heaven could not exist if Hell had not been created, and perfection, such as that promised by a utopian society, needs an enemy to contain the evil which must be disowned. Our liberal goals of a just world where hunger is solved by cooperation and wars are a thing of the past suffer from just that denial of the inevitable emergence of evil, especially in the form of envy and destructiveness. Relinquishing omnipotence is, then, a blow to the narcissistic belief that goodness can prevail, a phantasy that is difficult to give up.

2 These facts were: (1) the recognition 'of the breast as a supremely good object' on which the baby depends; (2) the recognition 'of the parental intercourse as a symbolic creative act' from which the infant is excluded because of its smallness and immaturity; and, finally, (3) the recognition 'of the inevitability of time and ultimately death' (Money-Kyrle, 1971, p. 443).

The reality principle does not demand that all omnipotent phantasy is given up, but insists that it can only be enjoyed as a daydream and not as an achievable goal. Unfortunately, the relegation of omnipotence to the world of the imagination requires a capacity for symbolic thinking, and giving up the lure of concrete solutions is never easy.

The question of how to let go of omnipotence is too important and too difficult to be addressed here, but it may just be worth mentioning Segal's insistence (1993) that before it can be given up, the pleasures of omnipotence need to be acknowledged. There is nothing quite as gratifying as the belief that we are the guardians of goodness over the evil of our enemies, and the pleasure of reversing humiliation with triumph can be irresistible. An awareness of the temptations of omnipotence can serve as a reminder to both patient and analyst that we are always trying to become master in our own house and that such mastery may create a fragile order which cannot survive contact with reality.

Chaos, Freedom, and Order in the Analytic Setting

The psychoanalyst confronts the need to balance the elements of chaos, freedom, and order when they attempt to define the optimum setting for conducting their work. They try to provide an environment in which order and stability can deliver freedom for the patient, and try to use order to reduce chaos without the threat of authoritarian rule. Of course, the patient may, and usually does, challenge boundaries and in doing so may threaten the safety of the setting and introduce chaos into it. At the same time, a degree of chaos needs to be tolerated if traditional dogmas are to be questioned and new patterns explored. Too much chaos feels unsafe, and too little chaos is over-restrictive and uncreative.

The Boundaries of the Setting

The boundaries are normally set by the analyst, who puts forward guidelines for issues such as session times, fees, holiday dates, the principle of paying for missed sessions, and the use of the couch, to which the patient is expected to give their assent. The most important aspect of the setting, however, is the adoption of a *psychoanalytic attitude*, which is what distinguishes psychoanalysis from other endeavours. The principal feature of the *analytic attitude* is the exclusive focus of the analyst's interest on the understanding of the patient, and to this end they try to avoid other activities such as providing advice and information. The demand for these other activities inevitably intrudes, and the patient may demand adjustments that force changes in the boundaries. The request for remote analysis is a good example of the need to explore the meaning of a change to the boundaries, while accepting the reality of the situation and attempting to retain the primary focus on understanding.

The Consent of the Governed

Looking for a model of just how freedom can be maximised, I turned to the American Declaration of Independence of 4 July 1776.[3]

> We hold these truths to be self-evident, that all men are created equal, that they are endowed by their Creator with certain unalienable Rights, that among these are Life, Liberty and the pursuit of Happiness. – That to secure these rights, Governments are instituted among Men, deriving their just powers from the consent of the governed.

Many of the issues that safeguard democracy are relevant to the analytic setting, perhaps the most important of which is the idea of government by consent. Normally the analyst's wish to sustain an analytic attitude is seen as the exercise of 'just powers', to which the patient agrees. But we are aware that the consent is not always forthcoming and may be viewed as a submission to power rather than jointly agreed. Sometimes the patient instals their own boundaries, which the analyst may be forced to accept, and mutual dissatisfactions with the way in which the analysis is conducted may threaten the stability of the setting. A patient experiencing resentments may make authoritarian demands and these in turn may provoke an authoritarian attitude in the analyst, making it more difficult to balance chaos, freedom, and order.

The Boundary Separating Order from Chaos

The need for a boundary to the setting that separates order from chaos is illustrated in the Book of Genesis, when God creates the Garden of Eden. In Milton's version (1674), the archangel Raphael explains to Adam how the world was created out of chaos.

> He took the golden Compasses, prepar'd
> In Gods Eternal store, to circumscribe
> This Universe, and all created things:
> One foot he center'd, and the other turn'd
> Round through the vast profunditie obscure,
> And said, thus farr extend, thus farr thy bounds,
> This be thy just Circumference, O World.
> (*Paradise Lost*, 7.225–231)

3 The full text can be found on the US National Archives website at: https://www.archives.gov/founding-docs/declaration-transcript.

This was how order was established in a circumscribed area within which man could flourish. An ideal environment of safety and freedom was ensured though the boundary that divided Eden from chaos and ultimately separated good from evil. Within Eden, life, liberty, and the pursuit of happiness were available to all, and the only rule that limited freedom was the injunction not to eat the fruit from the Tree of Knowledge. It is access to knowledge that distinguishes the Human from the Divine and limits freedom, just as children are protected from disturbing facts, especially those to do with sex and death. When the analyst chooses to keep some areas private the patient may feel excluded and provoked; withholding knowledge may be felt as evidence of a paternalistic system, which confers a superior position on the analyst. Some patients may then be strong enough to emulate Eve who, driven by curiosity, and encouraged by Satan, had the courage to break the taboo against knowledge and rebel against the limitation of her freedom to know. It is possible to think of her as the first rebel, whose courage sustained later explorers like Galileo and Darwin. Freud certainly thought of himself as a conquistador (Freud, 1900a).

Segal (2007) pointed out that even though it was claimed to be a disaster, the punishment for Adam and Eve acquiring knowledge was nothing more than to lose Paradise and live in the real world. God announced that henceforth Adam and Eve would have to work for their bread, Eve would suffer the pains of childbirth, and, most shocking, both would face the inevitability of death. In the real world the cost of freedom takes the form of suffering in accord with these facts of life, especially perhaps the reality of death. Our dreams of immortality are thus revealed as omnipotent phantasies, and the idealisation that creates the perfection of Paradise is seen to depend on ignorance and disappears when the forbidden knowledge is grasped. We are reminded of Lady Bracknell's pronouncement that 'Ignorance is like a delicate exotic fruit; touch it and the bloom is gone' (Oscar Wilde, *The Importance of Being Earnest*, Act 1).[4]

Like Eve, patients too must be willing to take risks if they are to explore the limits of what can be discovered in an analysis.

The Relationship between the Internal Parents

The super-ego is commonly referred to as if it were a unified object, but a closer view reveals it to be based on the internalisation of a parental couple in a complex relationship. The severity of paternal rule may or may not be moderated by maternal interventions, while the containing function of the mother may or may not be supported by the strength of the father.

Sometimes the couple become even more frightening than the single parent, and this seems especially so if they come to be entwined as a combined

4 The text can be accessed at https://www.gutenberg.org/files/844/844-h/844-h.htm.

parental object, usually combined in hatred of the child as well as of each other, as described by Klein (Steiner, 2017). If the child is to enlist the help of one parent against the tyranny of the other, the two parents must be capable of being divided before they can be tolerated as a couple.

Maternal Containment Functioning as an Exoskeleton

The anxieties created by uncontrolled id impulses and especially by fragmentation of the ego can be relieved if they are projected into the mother and integrated there through her capacity to give meaning to the projections. This mechanism, called containment by Bion (1962), enables the mother to provide an area of security and to create a boundary that separates order from chaos. Within this boundary the infant feels more whole and more secure, but rather as a mollusc depends on protection from its shell, its security is gained at the cost of freedom. The boundary aspects of the analytic setting have a similar containing function; they may provide safety but can lead to a claustrophobic fear of being trapped, like those patients of Henri Rey who saw the hospital as a brick mother.[5] In this way, maternal containment provides an exoskeleton that is an essential component of order, but for freedom to be established, it must be complemented with a form of internalised structure or backbone.

In order to escape from the restrictions of the exoskeleton, the organism evolved a spinal column, which enabled its descendants to gain their freedom and swim out into the open sea. Similarly, with the support of the internalised backbone, the infant can leave the mother's protection behind while still able to return to it if anxiety becomes too great. This is an enormous evolutionary step with huge advantages, perhaps best illustrated in the development of the toddler when it begins to walk. We see the excitement of its new-found freedom when the child takes its first steps, leaving the safety of its mother behind. Again, these liberating developments provide pleasure and confidence but can stimulate omnipotence unless restrained by the balancing containment of the maternal presence.

Excessive Chaos: Clinical Fragment, Ms A

I will look briefly at the situation of a patient whose life seemed to be dominated by chaos. She was in many ways competent but her affairs were in disarray and her appearance was dishevelled. She created an air of confusion in the sessions, and regularly muddled up her session times and holiday dates. The analyst was concerned by her self-neglect and puzzled by her mental confusion. She spoke slowly and was often silent and angry, as though she

5 Personal communication, 1966.

had all the time in the world, giving the impression that she had a secret source of richness and superiority beneath the chaos.

When the analyst tried to work with her and put some order into the sessions, she adamantly refused and created no-go areas that rendered any mention of the transference out of bounds. At the same time, she was distressed at her state, and would repeatedly complain that the analyst wasn't helping her.

In this analysis, chaos seemed to have the upper hand and left both the patient and the analyst confused and helpless. The analyst was devalued and abused as useless, as if the patient expected to be rescued from the chaos, perhaps by an idealised father or perhaps by a mother who would agree to clean up the messy child and make her lovable once more. The main casualty seemed to be the freedom to think, which was suppressed beneath a tyrannical determination to control the setting and prevent any joint work.

The analyst had to cope with her own confusion and helplessness and had to turn to internal sources of strength that enabled her to tolerate the chaos. Sometimes, the patient gave the impression of an adolescent refusing to tidy her room, and her negativity seemed to be supported by idealised phantasies that would have to be abandoned if she faced reality. A consideration of the balance between chaos, order, and freedom seemed to indicate that for both the patient and the analyst, freedom was the main casualty, and that chaos and attempts to create order through omnipotence dominated.

Excessive Order: Clinical Fragment, Mr B

Another patient, Mr B, seemed to suffer from an excessive need for order, which led him to create safety by keeping his distance. Soon after his analysis began, he accepted a post in another country, which obliged the analyst to accept a change to remote sessions. This kind of move had been characteristic of him ever since he had left his warring family to attend university. When he moved away, his wife also moved to a different city for work reasons; this situation left them only able to spend weekends and holidays together. Mr B lived by rigid rules that he deemed necessary but which he disliked; he felt they limited his emotional life. They had been established early in his childhood to regulate an over-intense entanglement with his mother, who had enlisted him as her ally in her battles against his father.

In one session, Mr B reported how he had felt obliged to agree when his wife proposed they have sex, and had ended up with a terrible headache, which forced him to stop. It made him feel sad and confirmed his inability to enjoy things.

The analyst also felt some regret that a lively and enjoyable session seemed out of bounds, and both were able to acknowledge the restricted contact without being able to do anything about it. Later, a similar limitation to what could be accomplished was discussed in relation to the tensions in Hong Kong; the patient felt he should have become involved in helping in some way because he had family connections there. He was also appalled at the arbitrary sackings of some colleagues at the hands of the Trump administration in the United States, but argued that he and his wife had been smart by always being ready to pack their bags and leave. His wife thought this was fine but he thought that always leaving areas of anxiety was cowardice, and he wished that someone would say, 'we are in this together and it is going to be OK'. This seemed an expression of his need for paternal support.

His fear of breaking rules was expressed when he cancelled a Friday session at the last minute and asked for a 'make-up' session. When he joined the session he was agitated, especially since the reason for the cancellation had been a holiday rather than work. He feared that he could be thrown out, and he remembered that he had once come to his session at the wrong time and had been sent away. At that time, he had been sure it was not his mistake, and he had sworn to himself that he would leave and never come back.

The analyst was able to pick up his fury at being made to feel in the wrong, which he felt as a humiliation and an exercise of her power. When he spoke openly and honestly to his wife about some of his worries, she had given him a hug, but he had felt it was simply dutiful and that they were only going through the motions of expressing feelings. He did not feel he deserved a hug and could take no pleasure from it because he could not allow himself to feel open and vulnerable. He explained that he did not have the right to be angry and mentioned that some years earlier, when he discovered his wife had had an affair, he had been so enraged that he stopped driving and got out of the car because he feared he might kill her. He had felt the same rage towards his mother when he felt he could not stand up to her. It might have been different if he were stronger or had someone to help him stay in contact.

Mr B's freedom to think, and especially to experiment and enjoy relationships, was limited by rigid rules that ensured that relationships remained intact but remote. He felt something was missing when he created a distance to ensure safety and was denied the pleasure and freedom that came from a lively interaction. Order was established at the cost of freedom, and he felt it was impossible for him to be master in his own house. The possibility of a warmer and deeper connection with an analyst who could survive his rage and help him to face the damage he felt he had done was a potential goal that evoked the earlier good relationship with a great-aunt, but which remained something for the future.

In this analysis, a longing for freedom was limited by rigid rules that produced a relationship that felt shallow and unreal. He desperately needed a paternal backbone, but he feared that masculine power was dangerous and had to be restrained by strict rules. He did seem to long for the freedom to express passionate feelings of both love and hate, but the rules meant that he could only go through the motions and was not able to risk a direct contact. It also seemed difficult for the analyst to express her feelings, in part because of her own rules, but also because he was so deeply wounded if he felt rejected.

It was very difficult for him to risk saying 'no' without also leaving the situation, and without this ability he could never be free. This meant that he could not tell his wife that he did not want sex or tell his analyst that he did not want a session, and he made it difficult for his analyst to defend her freedom to think and to discuss the parameters of the setting.

General Discussion

Freud's sympathy towards the poor ego can help us to understand how difficult it is for both the patient and the analyst to cope with the ego's three masters and to balance the forces of chaos, freedom, and order. It may also be difficult to understand which of these conditions should be given priority because we see how sometimes freedom is blocked by too much chaos, while at other times it is constrained by too much order. It is helpful to recognise that sometimes it is the fear of chaos that drives the ego into a collaboration with a severe super-ego to establish order. At other times, however, it is the fear of rebelling against a rigid organisation that limits the freedom to think and act against the rules.

In either case it is freedom that suffers; it can be thought of as the chief casualty of the conflict between chaos and order. Perhaps the idea of liberating the patient and the analyst to enjoy the freedom to think, even when such thinking seems to enter forbidden areas, can become a potential goal even if it seems to be a remote possibility. We must, however, also accept the limitations of our understanding, and we can at least agree with Freud (1933, p. 78) that 'Life is not easy!'

9 The Advantages and Disadvantages of Concrete Thinking

The Numbing Feeling of Reality[1]

Introduction

A consideration of Bion's 1961 paper on the numbing effect of reality allows me to re-examine his concept of containment. This important idea led Bion to the realisation that projective identification was an essential mechanism through which anxieties were relieved. His idea was that the infant, in a fragmented state, projects concrete elements of the self into the mother, who receives and integrates them, and through her understanding transforms them into symbolic elements. In his nomenclature, beta-elements are transformed by alpha-function into alpha-elements. The mother has to be in a receptive frame of mind called reverie, which Bion saw as a loose reticulum of thoughts that can give space to the child. If the mother's mind is preoccupied with some definite goal the projections are blocked, and the anxiety can be made worse. Bion spoke about a fear of death becoming a nameless dread.

In the ideal case, Bion suggests, the mother's capacity to symbolise is internalised and can be utilised by the child, but this seems to me to be a simplification of the process. A further step is required before the child can develop his own capacity to symbolise. Following a successful containment the mother is internalised, and it is her thinking that is utilised to relieve the anxiety. Before the child can develop his own symbolic function, the object has to be relinquished and mourned.

Bion's ideas about concrete thinking and concrete objects are explored in this chapter, which examines both the benefits and the costs of the change from the concrete to the symbolic. Bion called concrete objects beta-elements, which he saw as being projected into the mother and in optimal circumstances being contained and understood by her. Her capacity to symbolise, which he called alpha-function, could then be internalised and made use of by the child. This seems to describe the best-case scenario and even when these conditions are met, it commonly involves an internalisation at a concrete level, in that the alpha-function requires the continuing presence

1 This chapter is based on J. Steiner (2011b), The Numbing Feeling of Reality, *Psychoanalytic Quarterly*, 80: 73–89.

DOI: 10.4324/9781003726135-10

of the internal mother. It can be argued that to fully internalise the capacity to symbolise, the second step of relinquishing the mother and mourning her loss is required.

In his early paper on groups Bion described how the projection of concrete objects into the analyst is especially prone to take over the analyst's mind and paralyse his thinking. This is particularly likely to occur if there is an excessive emphasis on reality in the clinical material, which can numb the analyst's capacity to respond to projections. The numbing effect is enhanced when moral considerations support the patient's contention that his beliefs are entirely reasonable, and a double danger exists from the presence of both too much morality and too much reality.

I argue that in some circumstances, concrete thinking can be advantageous. For example, in times of war, perhaps, hostility to the enemy requires badness to be split off and attributed to others and symbolic function creates complications of feeling. At such times the analyst may have to accept the patient's concrete thinking but try to prevent becoming equally concrete himself.

In order to be receptive to the patient's needs the analyst has to remain independent but responsive to the unconscious communications from his patient. When anxiety is great and primitive mental mechanisms are employed, this can be difficult because the analyst is at the receiving end of projections which are concrete and disturbing. At such times the images are stripped of symbolic significance, and their intention is not so much to communicate as to pressure the analyst into playing a role in order to support the patient's defensive needs. It is particularly difficult to avoid giving in to such pressures if we are not aware that we have been taken over by the patient's projections and have been driven to enact rather than to understand. Without knowing it, we can become invaded by figures from the patient's internal world, whose existence in our own minds becomes so real that it diverts our attention from our relationship with the patient.

I describe how a preoccupation with the patient's reality and a submission to his morality can numb the analyst to an awareness of the psychic reality of the transference. In particular, this involves the reality of loss and a propensity by both patient and analyst to deny this through the deployment of omnipotent phantasy. When this is recognised by the analyst, he can adopt more limited and realistic goals and the omnipotence may gradually be relinquished and mourned.

In this chapter I am going to explore ways in which analyst and patient may become involved in repeated enactments and cycles of mutual projective identifications. I will try to show that this is particularly likely to create difficulties when the analyst does not recognise the concrete nature of the patient's projections into him and is drawn into playing the role of an object from the patient's internal world. Of course, a transient playing out of a role need not be thought of as a technical problem, and indeed is an essential component of the analyst's empathic understanding of the patient's position.

Ideally the analyst must allow himself to respond to projections and enactments, and in due course this may even enhance his understanding of both himself and of his patients. However he also has to be able to shake himself out of such an over-involvement and be able to return to a more receptive analytic stance.

The fact that this is not always easy arises from a combination of the analyst's personal vulnerabilities and the patient's use of projective identification, and these factors are clearly an inevitable part of the analytic relationship. The more the analyst can become aware of his propensity to succumb to the projections, the more he is in a position to extricate himself and once more to be receptive to underlying unconscious communications. However, to do so he may have to recognise the role played by his own defensive needs and to accept and mourn his own limitations.

I am going to describe two features in my patient's material that seemed to be particularly potent in paralysing an analytic attitude of free-floating attention. I came to characterise these as 'Too much reality and too much morality'. The patient repeatedly and vividly described cruel and unfair interactions in which he had felt enormous rage and to which I was exposed as a helpless observer. To him the unfairness was terribly real, and I felt pressured either to side with him or to challenge his view of things. I became drawn into the reality of his encounters and unable to remain open to the unconscious communications which lay beneath the descriptions. If I tried to be neutral or sceptical, I was made to feel that I disbelieved him and that I was allowing a terrible cruelty to proceed unnoticed.

I think Bion (1961, p. 149) may have had something similar in mind when, he suggested that normally it ought to be possible for the analyst to detect when his mind has been taken over. He described 'a distinct quality to the counter-transference that should enable [the analyst] to recognize that he is playing a role in somebody else's phantasy'. But he adds that this is sometimes difficult because of what he calls 'a temporary loss of insight, a sense of experiencing strong feelings and at the same time a belief that their existence is quite adequately justified by the objective situation without recourse to recondite explanation of their causation'.

The delusional quality of a belief may then come to be hidden by making it seem reasonable, and the analyst may either come to share it or to feel obliged to challenge it. Bion goes on to say: 'I believe [the] ability to shake oneself out of the numbing feeling of reality that is a concomitant of this state is the prime requisite of the analyst in the group' (Bion, 1961, p. 149).

The loss of insight arises from the way the patient is able to use projective identification to interfere with the capacity of the analyst to deploy symbols. While this is most extreme in the case of psychotic patients, lesser forms of such symbolic paralysis are common. Bion (1956, 1962), building on Segal's studies of symbolic function (Segal, 1954), proposed that in psychosis the capacity to symbolise is lost, and P. C. Sandler (1997) has usefully extended Bion's model by proposing that an anti-symbolic process operates to transform symbolic elements back into concrete objects. Bion argues that beta-elements are only suitable for projective identification since they cannot be symbolised, and I am raising the possibility here that the inverse is also true; namely, that in order to deploy projective identification effectively, a transformation from symbolic to concrete elements is necessary. When the patient's symbolic function is intact, meaningful connections are made to thoughts, memories, dreams, and other resonances in his life, and it is partly because of these connections that symbolic entities are difficult to get rid of by projective identification. They are also less potent in their effect on the analyst's mind than are their concrete counterparts. According to this idea, abstract symbolic elements have first to be converted back into a concrete form so that they can be got rid of by evacuation through projective identification.

I think it is likely that this type of reversal of symbolic capacity is an active process that operates widely, and which can also be used defensively by the analyst when he finds that he is unable to tolerate the symbolic implications of what has been projected into him. The adoption of an analytic stance may then create too much anxiety and guilt for it to be sustained, and concrete thinking becomes necessary for the analyst just as it was for the patient. The analyst may be driven by the experiences evoked in him to reverse his capacity to symbolise in order to transform the experience back into a concrete projectable form.

Usually this takes place at an unconscious level, and the projection takes the form of an enactment disguised as an interpretation. These interpretive enactments (Joseph, 2003; Steiner, 2006) subsequently make the analyst feel even more guilty and make it very difficult for them to recognise what is happening in order to extricate themselves from behaviour which for a time seems no different from the patient's.

From a broader point of view, we can see that the reversal of symbolic capacity is a necessary mechanism to relieve the individual of unbearable mental experiences, whether they are a patient or an analyst. Without it, projective identification would be impossible and our defensive organisation would not be able to function. If the analyst can resist some of the pressure to enact and retain a capacity to think, they may be able to recognise a meaningful communication underlying the projections. The analyst may then become aware of the patient's need to project and be in a position to help the patient to feel understood. Bion's observations, which I believe were corroborated in the work I am going to present, suggest that containment is made more difficult if there is too much reality accompanying the patient's projections. The analyst is persuaded that the emotions they feel are justified by the reality of the situation, and does not realise that they are being taken over by the projection onto them of an object from the patient's internal world. To receive, contain, and understand the projections, the analyst has to be able to shake themselves out of the numbing feeling of reality. They can then sometimes recognise that they are being influenced to behave not like a psychoanalyst but like one of the patient's internal objects or like the patient themselves.

Clinical Material

This theme was specifically raised in the analysis of a patient who was able to draw me into a preoccupation with the concrete issues he was obsessed with. These issues were terribly real to him, and they frequently became real to me. I was numbed, almost hypnotised, and could not prevent myself from engaging at a concrete level. I behaved as if I believed that I could sort out what was 'really' happening in the patient's life. This meant that I vacated my position of free-floating attention and that I became numb to the deeper and more meaningful communications. At the time of writing the paper on which this chapter is based, I was growing more aware of this problem, and in the material I present I was sometimes able to interpret his unconscious wishes and needs, for example that we each face our helplessness and recognise our excursions into omnipotence. However, it is also clear that for much of the time I behaved as if I could protect him from persecution and even persuade him to behave in a less omnipotent way. His capacity to engage me in his concrete situation dovetailed with my own defensive needs and created the numbing situation that I am trying to describe.

The patient chiefly spoke about his life at home and sometimes about his career, both of which seemed to be in a perpetual crisis. His relationship with his mother had been difficult since the death of his father some ten years previously, and before my Christmas break, the relationship had deteriorated so much that he temporarily moved out of the family home. Highly charged accounts of verbal attacks from his mother filled many sessions, while his search for a job, by contrast, was mostly characterised by a lack of anxiety and an unconvincing optimism. For the patient, both situations were terribly real and evoked strong feelings that seemed entirely to be justified by his circumstances. But for the analyst, they were so dramatised that it was impossible to be clear about what was really going on. I was pulled from side to side in my reactions to his domestic crises, sometimes feeling that his mother was entirely reasonable, while at other times feeling that he was justified in his complaints against her.

Session One

In the first session after a Christmas break, the patient began by saying that the gap had seemed much longer than a fortnight. His experience of this time could only be described as unremitting hell. He then gave a detailed account of the crisis which had arisen after his aunt had been diagnosed with cancer. 'Actually', he said, 'it is much worse than that. The situation was dire. Not only was she suffering terribly but no one was helping.' His aunt would phone his mother at four in the morning, pouring out her suffering, and his mother would then turn on the patient and attack him for his inability to help. He then described his own efforts to intervene to help his aunt, and how his plan to rally support from his uncles and other men in the family had met with rejection and apathy, and far from being appreciated, had increased the attacks made on him.

Next, he explained that he had woken a week previously with pain in his abdomen. The GP had said it was an infection, but it had not improved with antibiotics. 'It is apposite', he said, 'I feel kicked in the guts.' He continued, 'What else might interest you? My mum has said that a room in the house will be available, and largely because of your influence I elected to claim it as mine. So the plan is that I move back into the house this evening, although, in fact, I have been spending most of my time there in the holidays. What a waste of money the temporary flat was. And it has been hell. I know that, and you know that. My aunt got much worse. It was awful. I expect you have had quite a nice Christmas. You wouldn't trade it for mine, and I don't blame you.'

I interpreted that he wanted me to know that I had left him in an awful state. Like the men in the family, I had failed to be available, and this had left him looking after everyone else and feeling that his needs, and even his health, were neglected. I was meant to see how dire it was, and to imagine the possibility that he too might have cancer, while I enjoyed good health and enjoyable holidays.

He went on to suggest that it had been a stupid idea to think that the men in the family would help. 'But it was interesting. It clarified what my family was like. I make all the effort and they make no concessions. I can't even have a rest. They have no guts. Stupid people dominated by a bunch of horrendous witches.'

I responded by saying that he was trying to challenge me to see if I could take on these awful accusations, or was I going to claim that I had behaved responsibly and had left him well cared for? He was frightened that like everyone else I could not tolerate guilt and responsibility and would make out that he was to blame.

He said it was clear that he could expect nothing. It had been naïve, quixotic, to think the men could help, and he should have known better:

'What good will rearranging rooms do? It is ridiculous. Today I am going to the library where it is peaceful, for a rest.'

I interpreted that he wanted me to know that he could not see the point of having a room of his own, and at the moment he did not want a space of his own to be able to think. He was relieved that he was coming to his session, where, like the library, it was more peaceful because I did not attack him and he could hand over his thinking to me.

'So?', he said. 'Nothing is any different, but just as usual. In my family everything is a trap. I avoid most of them but I cannot avoid them all.'

Discussion of Session One

The patient tried to convey to me what an unremitting hell he had gone through, and to a degree did succeed in making me feel guilty. Responsibility and guilt over his situation, just like that for his aunt's cancer, was passed on from person to person. The aunt phoned his mother at 4 a.m. His mother listened and then railed against the patient, who in turn used the session to project the guilt into me. The patient accepted his aunt's behaviour as reasonable, and in view of her distress his mother's attack on him also seemed reasonable. To suggest that anyone was being dramatic and unreasonable was morally unacceptable.

I think one version of his psychic reality was that the patient was left to cope with all the projections coming at him from every direction and the hell this created felt like a kick in the guts, leaving him in pain that was being neglected by a preoccupied analyst. Responsibility for the suffering of others was projected into him, and his narcissism allowed him to accept this, even though he could not live up to the expectation that he would put it right. Both the moral pressure put on him and the apparent reality of the suffering were persuasive, and in the sessions it was these pressures that seemed to draw me into a similar adoption of responsibility and guilt that encouraged omnipotence. To retain an analytic attitude, I had to accept his suffering and to feel the pain of my inability to help him. If I could understand his need to project his guilt and responsibility into me, I was more able to avoid seeking relief from this pain by attempting to rescue him from his unhappy situation.

The patient did ask his mother for the newly available room and had arranged to occupy it when he returned home. Now, however, in his rage he was making it clear that the symbolic connection with a space in his mind where he could think was of no use to him. He needed to evacuate the pain and distress, and thinking would be an impediment that made projection more difficult. This meant that I had to try to preserve a capacity to think without expecting him to join me in a symbolic discourse, which he was not at that moment capable of.

The difficulty of containment was evident when I failed to resist his demand that I was to find concrete solutions to his predicament, and this led me to become embroiled in his version of reality. At those times, I was unable to retain an analytic attitude of receptivity to the unconscious communications that I later came to think might have involved a dread of separateness and loss. I felt I had been acting out, and this left me feeling dissatisfied and incompetent. When thinking about it afterwards I felt that something had paralysed my thinking, and I wondered if this was an instance of Bion's notion of 'the numbing sense of reality'. Was this why I could not see beyond the repetitive issues of his cruelty to his mother or her cruelty to him? His account of what happened was on the one hand so real and on the other so dramatised that, at a factual level, it was impossible to know what to believe. Nevertheless, I felt a need to evaluate his reality and to decide whether he was a victim or a perpetrator of the particular injustice he was occupied with. I tried to avoid making judgemental interpretations, but it was often difficult not to take sides, and a critical tone was difficult to keep out of my interpretations.

In my defence, I did think that sometimes he was able to feel and to communicate some real pain and I often felt he had some insight into the way a quite awful suffering was being played out before us, as if we were both observers of a soap opera. This led to some contact with depression and mental pain, even though it felt once removed, and I sometimes wondered if he was not in this way communicating his helplessness as well as acknowledging mine.

Periodically, it was possible to discern a shift in the mood of the sessions, when the patient was quieter and more reflective. It was difficult to know what led to this change but sometimes at least, it seemed to follow a recognition on my part that I had been trying too hard and had not been able to face my helplessness. Some evidence of this could be discerned in a session which took place before the next break, in which the same noisy complaints of injustice and cruelty were present, but a new note of sadness was also discernible.

Session Two

The patient began the session describing another extremely dramatic, disturbing, and intense row with his mother. This had followed a meeting between his mother and his sister in which they had got together and made defamatory accusations about him that confirmed his status as unwanted and unloved in his family. Both his sister and his mother had adopted the role of victim, and when they blamed him for everything he argued that they must be right. He spoke about his mother's 'incredible suffering', which he could do nothing to relieve, and how he simply became furious and aggrieved. The account went on for a long time without any reference to his analysis or to the fact that in three days I was to embark on my Easter break.

Most of this was quite familiar, but on a somewhat sadder note he said that he could see no alternative for his life but to keep things as they were, waiting for the dire outcome when it came. He thought his mother would probably wait until after her holiday in the summer and then throw him out. A sensible person would prepare and find a flat for himself, but he knew that he would just wait and see what happened. In the meantime he would do his best to be patient and supportive.

I interpreted that he knew that in a few days I was going to be away and he felt that both he and I were helpless to alter this. Instead of facing our helplessness, we were caught in an atmosphere of blame in which everyone felt themselves to be a victim and blamed everyone else. He said that he did not agree: he was simply describing what had happened that morning. I pointed out the dramatic way in which he had talked about his mother's 'incredible suffering', which I thought was how he felt about his own suffering. I suggested that the purpose of the dramatic accusations and counter-accusations was to make me recognise that I was leaving him in a hopeless situation. He replied that the only thing he was clear about was his fury, but he added that he still had the fantasy that his mother would change. She would realise what she was doing to him.

I interpreted that he really did hope that I would reconsider and cancel my break, or agree to take him with me. If his cries and protests made me relent, then the hell he was living in would be transformed into a heaven. He let out a laugh of ridicule at this idea, and I interpreted that he was mocking anything childish or needy in himself, because all he could envisage was to be rescued and this did not seem real. However I suggested that his feelings were real and were leading him to go on trying to get relief. If he could make me feel bad about the state I was leaving him in, he might at least feel that a measure of his suffering had got through to me.

He said that he had stopped talking about his career problems, and his mother behaved as if they had disappeared. She accused him of exploiting her and his sister, using their money to finance his easy life, and that it was now time he paid them back what he owed. I interpreted that he felt he was the one who was being exploited, including in the way I seemed able to take my break with no regard for him. Yet I also suggested that it was impossible to tell what the reality was. Was he really suffering or was he getting satisfaction from the drama that was playing out in front of me? Perhaps if the drama stopped he would be faced with the emptiness and deadness that my absence would leave him with.

He paused and then described how he had put his arm around his mother's shoulder and she had rejected him, accusing him of insensitivity. Her sister was dying and all he could offer her was a hug. I interpreted that he felt that my attempts to support and comfort him were inadequate. He wanted material help not understanding. His situation was made worse by my ability to leave while he was stuck in his dire situation. I had a way out. I was sufficiently together to be able to afford a break and what was more, to him this heralded the eventual end of the analysis. I would be able to retire and extricate myself, and he could find no such option. 'Yes', he said, 'you are in a position to think of retirement because you have the means to do so while I have nothing.'

I said that I was meant to believe that I would be leaving him with nothing and yet it was difficult for me to tell what his resources were. Nor were mine so clear to him, although he preferred to think of me in terms of clichés of having an easy life, being happy and successful, a situation which he wanted for himself, and felt deprived of. 'Yes', he said, 'but of course, it is possible that you are going through some dire situation like the one my aunt is in.'

Discussion of Session Two

This session began with the familiar dramatic accounts of blame and counter-blame, in which moral issues were so dominant that the reality could not be evaluated. I thought my patient felt that my break was bitterly unfair and cruel, and that it made him feel like a child left with few resources while the parents callously went off to the adult world with its emotional and material riches. Instead of understanding this and supporting his experience of a deeply immoral world, I was questioning his version of reality, and, like his mother and sister, was implying that he owed me something, while he felt that it was me who owed him. In this way I became drawn into a struggle to get rid of guilt. I think he felt I could not bear to face my responsibility for misunderstanding him and was implying that he was to blame for the way he was dramatising events in his life in order to make me feel bad. He felt that I was trying to blame him, although it was me who deserved to feel bad since I was the one leaving him. He felt that I was not able to accept the emotional reality which underlay his protests.

At this stage of the session, all the parties involved seemed to be claiming that they were victims, and I think he found it very confusing. When he became angry at least he knew where he was, but in his rage there was no room for thinking or understanding. I think he felt more understood after he expressed his helplessness in the face of being thrown out by his mother. I was able to take up his despair that nothing could change and that all he could do was to hang onto his analysis, just as he would hang onto his mother, waiting for the dire outcome. At one level this could also be seen as trying to project guilt, but I thought it was associated with a sad mood arising from the recognition that he would eventually have to face losing his good objects. This theme was associated with the idea that I had a way out; I had enough resources – both emotional and material – to escape, while he felt trapped. With this patient there was always the idea of a catastrophe in the background. He had spoken about having no exit policy, and it made me fear that if nothing changed we would have to face a collapse, leading to a breakdown.

Often the idea of a breakdown was simply unthinkable, but on this occasion it was associated with a sadder and more despairing mood. My own feelings of sadness were accentuated when he expressed the hope that his mother might change and finally realise what she was doing to him. He knew that I would not change my plans and cancel my break or take him with me, but he could express these longings as a small child might do, and I could respond with an awareness that I could comfort him perhaps, but that I was helpless to relieve his pain.

The view that understanding was inadequate was conveyed by his mother's dissatisfaction when he had put his arm around her shoulder. He asked himself if he had been doing something unreasonable by trying to comfort her. I think he was also confused by my efforts to support him through an understanding of his plight while not being able to relieve it. This brought us back to what he felt was the terrible difference in our circumstances. I could get away. I had an exit strategy associated with an eventual end to his analysis in which I was able to retire, while he was left with no way out.

The Role of Reality in Mourning

The contact with feelings of sadness and loss was associated with a capacity to think that involved the use of symbols proper (alpha-function), which enabled the patient, at least transiently, to feel understood. Thinking involved facing loss, made acute by the break but connected with the idea of losing me permanently. Were it to be fully faced, the loss would have to be accepted and mourned, and this was clearly only possible for a short time. Once he had experienced the pain and despair, he felt that he would need material relief rather than understanding. Just as he saw no point in having a room of his own in the first session, he saw my understanding in the second as representing an arm around his shoulder that was insufficient and confusing. He could not relinquish the hope that I would change my mind and be able to give him material rather than symbolic relief. Symbolic thinking was converted back into a concrete demand that the loss be reversed and his suffering transformed rather than understood. In this way his hell would be transformed into a heaven and both he and his objects would be omnipotently restored.

Gradually, over the course of the analysis, his capacity to sustain contact with sadness and loss had strengthened, and it seemed to me possible that it would continue to do so. This contact was associated with mourning, and with mourning came the capacity to take back some of the projections that had dominated so much of his analysis (Steiner, 1996a). Evidence of this capacity could sometimes be discerned in the patient, and he did finally moderate some of the extreme images of heaven and hell which reflected the contrast he felt between his situation and mine. However it was perhaps more important to discover in me the same capacity to sustain contact, and this involved a recognition of my difficulty in facing the loss of my patient and with it the loss of my sense of therapeutic potency. This brought me up against a consideration of the reality of what could and what could not be achieved in this analysis and through analysis in general. These limitations needed to be faced and worked through – eventually by the patient, but perhaps initially by the analyst. Mourning played a critical role in this process, and was ultimately not just for the loss of objects on which we depend but also for the loss of omnipotence on the part of both analyst and patient. If omnipotent solutions are relinquished, a potential for development can be released but of course such development is uncertain, gradual, partial, and slow.

Development of symbolic function (alpha-function) and the capacity to mourn are inextricably linked but often seem to give rise to a catch-22 situation. You can't mourn unless you can symbolise, and you can't acquire symbolic function unless you can mourn. If loss is felt to be unacceptable, then the experience has to be got rid of, and symbols need to be converted back into concrete objects so that relief can be obtained via projective identification. If the analyst is also unable to tolerate loss, it affects their capacity to contain so that there may be no one able to symbolise, tolerate the loss, and mourn it.

Much of the pressure on the analyst came from the patient's need for the analyst to clarify whether he was a good or a bad object. This stemmed in part from the patient's confusion and from his fear of becoming dependent on an unreliable object. It was increased by the conviction that he could not make these judgements himself. He believed that he was dependent on the analyst's judgements, while at the same time feeling that these were not to be trusted. As long as this situation continued, symbolic equivalents (beta-elements) were the primary means of communication, and the development of the patient's capacity to think and to symbolise was delayed.

An essential step in this development comes from acquiring a space to think and what Britton (2018) calls an emancipation of the ego from a dominance by the super-ego. I see this to mean that ego functions, in particular a capacity to evaluate and tolerate reality, come to be less dominated by super-ego functions which give priority to moral issues. We have to be able to tolerate what is and distinguish it from what should be. This task, I believe, involves a process of mourning and the replacement of a phantasied omnipotence with a capacity to make painful judgements, often specifically on what is real and what is delusional.

Much of the patient's dependence on omnipotence stemmed from his experience of reproachful objects who demanded that they be restored and repaired. Moreover, this repair had to be concrete because the patient could not understand the idea of symbolic reparation. What was disturbing was that for much of the time, neither could I. I saw him as damaged, and I felt guilty that I could not concretely restore him to health. A shift in my attitude required that I recognise the same painful helplessness in relation to my own internal world. Like him I wanted to restore and repair my damaged objects, and like him I failed to recognise that this can only be done symbolically.

In our profession it is particularly easy for us to project our own internal objects into our patients and then try to restore them by attempting to cure the patient. To recognise this as omnipotent involves letting our objects go and mourning them, and at the same time letting our omnipotence go and mourning it. If the analyst can see that their apperception of reality has been numbed, they can sometimes also see that they have become invaded by the patient's reality and have accepted a morality that was based on a concrete need to repair rather than to understand.

Often the central issue turns out to revolve around the experience of loss and the evaluation of the reversibility or otherwise of the loss. Freud was clear when he described how 'Each single one of the memories and situations of expectancy which demonstrate the libido's attachment to the lost object is met by the verdict of reality that the object no longer exists' (1917b, p. 255). To accept the loss as real involves a challenge to omnipotence when we have to admit that the loss cannot be reversed. It is also a challenge to our morality when we are forced to observe suffering which we believe ought to be prevented. It sometimes seems to be paradoxical that the way to help both the patient and the analyst to face the verdict of reality involves a detachment from the patient's versions of both morality and reality.

Strachey made a similar point when he emphasised that to make a mutative interpretation, the analyst has to eschew

> any real behaviour that is likely to confirm the patient's view of him as a 'bad' or a 'good' phantasy object. ... It is a paradoxical fact that the best way of ensuring that [the patient's] ego shall be able to distinguish between phantasy and reality is to withhold reality from him as much as possible. (Strachey, 1934, pp. 146–147)

In the case I have discussed, the patient provoked a constant preoccupation on my part with his reality, as if I felt obliged to decide whether I should believe him or not. In retrospect it is clear that this was the wrong question. Perhaps I might have followed the suggestion made by Bion that we could imagine the patient was reporting a dream rather a real event. Say that my patient had reported a dream in which his mother had attacked him unfairly. Perhaps this might have enabled me to extricate myself from issues of what was real and to respond to the patient's material as a communication of a symbolic kind, involving my capacity to face his and my own psychic reality.

I have found that looking at the role played by reality has allowed me to rethink my propensity to become preoccupied with the reality of patients' accounts and hence to miss the psychic reality which is being communicated. I doubt if it will stop me from indulging in enactments for defensive reasons, but perhaps it will allow me to study what has been enacted in a more tolerant way.

10 Acquiring a Personal Identity[1]

Introduction

Both a tribal identity and a personal identity are important, but breaking away from the parents represents an important move towards individual freedom of thought and inevitably demands facing conflict. Indeed, finding a mind of one's own (Numa, 2023) is unconsciously experienced as a murder of the parents and, in keeping with themes from the other chapters of this book, mourning plays a central role. It is argued that facing the guilt of the Oedipal crime and mourning the loss of the parents is the price that has to be paid for separateness.

Perhaps the most important contribution psychoanalysis can make to the understanding of identity is to explore its dependence on our relationship to internal objects. To a significant degree we gain an identity through identifications with the primary objects of infancy, and gradually with other significant parental figures as we grow up. Later these are extended to prominent figures in society and in literature and myth. In this way we gain an identity from a family, school, nation, religion, profession, gender, or race. The ability to announce 'I am an Englishman', 'a Christian', or 'a Socialist', can create a sense of belonging and communicate a set of values that help to answer the question, 'Who am I?'

However, a wish to discover a personal identity separate from that of the parents is part of a drive towards separation and individuation in development. When successful, this leads to a personal identity based on an internal self, separate from but in a relationship with internal parents. However, the situation is complicated because the wish to be separate is in conflict with the wish to cling on, and the process of separation is obstructed through the operation of defence mechanisms that prevent change. In particular, introjective and projective identifications lead to self and object becoming entangled

1 Based on J. Steiner (2023a), 'Foreword', in Numa (2023): a book written by members of my postgraduate workshop on the topic of identity.

DOI: 10.4324/9781003726135-11

with each other so that neither of them is able to relinquish possession of the other and both are distorted and misrepresented.

Nevertheless, a degree of separateness between self and object usually emerges because the identifications are normally flexible and reversible. This enables the individual to accept both an identity as an individual and retain their membership of the family and social group.

Sometimes however, separateness is firmly resisted, and the composite-object becomes difficult to unpack. It is then not possible to sort out what belongs to self and what belongs to the object, and a personal identity separate from that of the group fails to emerge. In these cases, the object is possessed and distorted by introjective and projective identifications and exists in the internal world as a concrete body not properly differentiated from the self.

Generational Change

The evolution of personal identity begins early in development and continues throughout life. Separateness is linked with sleeping alone, going to school, and forming peer groups; a critical moment that epitomises the process takes place when, as young adults, we leave home to establish a new family of our own. Here the conflict between individuation and possession becomes stark and unavoidable because a breakaway from dependent ties on the parents is required for a new family to be established. Other steps in adult life, which involve the capacity to think independently while simultaneously being rooted in developments in the past, make true independence possible. Creative developments in various fields of endeavour and new discoveries in science, literature, and art require both a dependence on the old and a willingness to overthrow previous dogmas.

An important indicator of an independent personal identity lies in the individual's creative capacity, which comes to represent the successful espousal of the new over the old. This aspect of identity is nicely stated in the biblical phrase, 'Ye shall know them by their fruits' (Matthew 7:16, KJV), which implies that our identity is reflected in our actions. Creativity above all requires a move from our primary objects to those in our own generation, and a break from the family is necessary, even if it is painful and frightening. Indeed in unconscious phantasy such a break is experienced as an Oedipal murder, and when the murder is taken seriously the consequences have to be faced. The overthrow of the parents leads to feelings of anxiety and loss, but also to feelings of regret, remorse, and guilt, which can release loving feelings and a wish to make reparation. After a successful rebellion, the working though of the mourning for the lost parents restores the relationship with them, now as objects separate from the self. Creativity depends on the capacity to symbolise, and that capacity depends on the capacity to mourn: to move from the concrete possession of the actual object to a relationship with a symbolic representative of it.

The Emancipation of the Ego from the Dominance of the Super-Ego

An important quality that is commonly assigned to parental figures is the function of judgement itself. The super-ego can be seen as the agency that sets standards of excellence by which we are judged but it acquires severity when it also acts as a judge of how these standards have been met. Britton (2018) pointed out that making judgements is an ego function through which we evaluate the state of things as they are. When usurped by the super-ego, the capacity to judge acquires a moralistic connotation, which is concerned with what 'should be' rather than 'what is'. If the patient can 'emancipate' their ego from dominance by the super-ego, they can begin to weigh up their own decisions and even pass judgement on their super-ego figures. Good and bad elements in ourselves and our parents become discernible so that we can identify with aspects we value and oppose those we disagree with. It is this differentiation that is so difficult when unconscious projective and introjective identifications distort what belongs to self and object. Following Strachey (1934), we can recognise that an important goal of analysis is to modify the severity of the super-ego, but Britton's approach helps us to see that it is sometimes just as important for the patient to be able to stand up to a tyrannical super-ego.

True and False Identities

All such developments involve the risk of conflict with powerful internal and external objects, and at times may create a gap between a private view of ourselves and a mask or public persona behind which we need to hide. Winnicott (1965), for example, has described a true self that more directly expresses wishes and desires but which is hidden beneath a false self, presented in deference to external opinion. These conflicts may weaken confidence in a personal identity that depends on the integrity of the ego, especially when the gap between the two identities is not recognised. Multiple identities, such as those seen in 'as-if' personalities, or even in impostors, may result (Deutsch, 1955). On the other hand, we all have hidden secret parts of the self that we know about but may not wish to show to the world. If we recognise that secret identities are universal, it is easier to respect our patient's and our own wish to exercise a right to privacy. The poet Elizabeth Bishop refused to speak about her sexuality in public, asserting that she relied on, 'closets, closets and more closets' (Tóibín, 2015).

The Critical Role of Mourning in the Establishment of Separateness

We have seen that the drive to individuation is thwarted unless, at least in phantasy, a violent break from the dominance of internal super-ego figures is undertaken. Sometimes this requires heroic actions in which omnipotence plays a part and the cost is often high. When the violence subsides and a return to reality is established, we become aware that the figures we hated and had to escape from are also the figures we loved and valued. The damage done becomes apparent and gives rise to regret, remorse, and guilt. It is these feelings that make us aware of our love and that can lead to moves towards reparation.

It is the process of working through such losses, accepting responsibility for them, and mourning them that enables projections previously attributed to objects to be returned to the self (Steiner, 1996a). Freud described how, in the work of mourning (1917b), each memory of the lost object is taken out and the verdict of reality applied to it. This verdict separates what is alive from what is dead, what can be retained and what is lost, and it enables elements of the self previously projected into the object to be returned to the ego. In this way, the ego is strengthened and the object becomes less distorted. These changes help to establish a personal identity based on a stronger ego while establishing internal relationships with less distorted super-ego figures.

The Conflict between Holding On and Letting Go of Primary Objects

The anxiety created by the move towards independence can be so threatening that powerful defences are deployed that retain a possessive hold to prevent loss and to control and limit the freedom of the object. Projective and introjective identifications are again deployed to recreate an amalgam of self and object that is resistant to change. These types of object relationships have been studied under the heading of Narcissistic Organisations, especially by Rosenfeld (1971), and involve mechanisms using power such as those described by Freud as a drive for mastery (Freud, 1905). This theme has been studied by French analysts (Laplanche and Pontalis, 1967; Denis, 1997); among these, Dorey (1986) has made a detailed examination of power relations, which he found were particularly prominent in perverse and obsessional patients. In the perverse type, sexual excitement plays a critical role and sado-masochistic phantasies cruelly imprison the object. In the obsessional type, phantasies of anal control set up an alternation between possession and release, leading to cruelty which repeatedly needs to be undone and checked. Introjective and projective identifications with bad objects can lead to an idealisation of power, which is felt to be stronger than love, and can become ego-syntonic and be established as a character trait.

The issue of mastery is also relevant to the object relations seen in melancholia, in which a damaged or dying object is identified with and possessed. Freud described how the object then casts its shadow on the ego, and separateness is prevented unless it can be relinquished and mourned.

Finally, I will briefly mention the importance of irony in the appraisal of identity. The ability to entertain doubts, avoid grandiosity, and laugh at one's pretensions requires a capacity to stand back and view oneself dispassionately. Taking an ironic view means that we can entertain more than one view of ourselves and smile at the contradictions that emerge. This makes us less rigid and also more tolerant of others. Identity itself has long-term implications and does not change from moment to moment, but our view of ourselves may sometimes change dramatically, so that we can feel successful sometimes and then plunge into a depression following a disappointment. It is irony that helps to support both views, as we admit that we cannot always sustain the image of ourselves that we would like to have. Similarly, the dependence on both tradition and innovation means that we sometimes adopt the identity of family, nation, or religion and then realise that we actually have independent views that shape our identity. An ironic stance is difficult to sustain if object relations are concrete and self and object are confused, as in the pathological organisations discussed above. When the object is more separate, symbolic function is facilitated, and with it irony becomes possible.

11 The Impostor Revisited[1]

Introduction

This chapter consists of a paper (Steiner, 2011c) commissioned to commemorate two classical papers on impostors by Phyllis Greenacre and Helene Deutsch. Both of these eminent American psychoanalysts felt impostors to be common among our patients, but also in our colleagues and within ourselves.

We all seek admiration and external validation of our worth, and we may feel that what we claim to be is a fraudulent, borrowed identity that is not our own. This includes our professional identity, since we profess to be psychoanalysts but feel we are impostors when we cannot live up to this claim.

It is no easy task to accept our imperfections without undermining the sense of identity which must of necessity accommodate feelings of self-doubt and guilt. Again, it is important to stress the relevance of mourning in the creation of a stable sense of self separate from that of the parents.

Phyllis Greenacre begins her classic paper by reminding us that 'An impostor is not only a liar, but a very special type of liar who *imposes* on others fabrications of his attainments, position, or worldly possessions' (1958b, p. 359; 2011, p. 1025). Yet she also recognises a wide range of conditions which bear a resemblance to that of the impostor, and she observes that the analyst 'quite frequently gets glimpses of such traits' in patients who are otherwise not overtly dishonest (1958b, p. 360; 2011, p. 1026).

Helene Deutsch (1955) is even more explicit about the ubiquity of variants of this condition, and clearly sees the impostor on a continuum that includes the 'as-if' personality of her earlier descriptions. She writes:

> The world is crowded with 'as-if' personalities, and even more so with impostors and pretenders. Ever since I became interested in the impostor, he pursues me everywhere. I find him among my friends and acquaintances, as well as in myself. (Deutsch, 1955, p. 1022)

1 Based on J. Steiner (2011c), 'The Impostor Revisited', *Psychoanalytic Quarterly*, *80*: 1061–1071.

DOI: 10.4324/9781003726135-12

The authors agree that we are all impostors to varying degrees, and even suggest that talented individuals, especially artists, may be particularly susceptible to feelings of fraudulence. Along the same continuum are patients who hide their true self within a false self (Winnicott, 1965) and those who defensively adopt a 'character armour' (Reich, 1933). These papers are therefore important not only in the understanding of these interesting patients but in understanding the impostor element in all of our patients as well as in ourselves. They are also a step towards the understanding of how it is that a sense of personal identity develops. The papers were of special interest to me because of my work with patients who hide in a psychic retreat, protected by a narcissistic organisation (Steiner, 1993a, 1993b; 2011c).

I was impressed with the special expertise that both authors brought to bear on the problem of the impostor. Deutsch was able to make links with her earlier classic work on patients with an 'as-if' personality (1942), her studies of female sexuality (1925), and her papers on *folie à deux* collusions and the family romance (1938). Greenacre made links with her work on psychopathic personalities (1952) and on the biological origins of a sense of identity (1958a). She has also written on the family romance of the artist (1958b) and on the relation of the impostor to the artist (1958c). Both authors looked beyond the specific and unusual features of their patients and recognised the universality of the problem.

Greenacre felt that she could not present analytic material because of problems of confidentiality, and these patients clearly present special difficulties over and above those we all struggle with. Instead, she discussed famous impostors from biographies and also made many pertinent observations from what is clearly a considerable clinical experience. Deutsch also drew on her vast experience, making many general observations as well as describing a patient in detail.

Factors in the Creation of the Impostor

Both Deutsch and Greenacre recognise the importance of pathological narcissism, and they are very aware that the impostor depends on their audience. Indeed, sometimes they are led to admire the skill with which the impostor enlists the observer to join them in their deception. Sometimes the observer has their own agenda for colluding with the impostor, as for example in the story of the Emperor's new clothes, where the admiring audience saw through the narcissism but for reasons of their own went along with it and flattered the Emperor.

The authors agree that a false self or 'as-if' personality is not sufficient to define the impostor. Additional features are required; the authors suggest that an excitement, often arising from an Oedipal triumph, fuels the deception. The excitement and narcissistic gratification which arises from the capacity to dupe an audience functions as a defence against the infant's sense of smallness and helplessness. This helplessness is transformed into a narcissistic superiority through identification with powerful objects, and the success of the identification is supported by the encouragement of an accomplice. Both the authors see this as representing an Oedipal triumph in which, with the support of the mother, the father is defeated.

Another issue which is prominent in both accounts is the failure of the superego to create a climate in which reality can be faced. Deutsch speaks of her patient's bloated ego ideal, and both authors recognise that part of the achievement of the impostor is to foster a belief that they have achieved their ego ideal. There is then no conflict between their actual self and what their ideal self might be.

Self-doubt, as Greenacre suggests, may be particularly characteristic of creative artists, who present a work of art for the judgement of others. It may then require enormous internal strength to retain a sense of one's worth if that work is not supported by the admiration of others. The case of the artist represents a paradox, since not only do they have a propensity to become an impostor, but their creative work requires a contact with reality that often demands honesty and strength. I will discuss this issue in the case of Leonardo da Vinci later in the chapter.

Looking at these papers more than 50 years on and from a transatlantic Kleinian perspective. I am impressed by the depth and subtlety of these experienced and sensitive clinicians. In a schematic way I will describe our current approach to identifications, both introjective and projective identifications, and discuss how these may lead to disorders of personal identity. I will describe the importance of the idea of an internal world to Kleinian analysts and how internal objects are constantly being projected onto figures in the external world, and re-introjected, sometimes modified by the experience. A critical issue in the genesis of an impostor arises when their objects are unable to contain and understand what is projected into them, and instead are drawn into enactments of various kinds. If the patient can recognise the analyst's limitations, it helps the patient to think about their own. For both, it is often the relinquishment of omnipotence that is most resisted, and when it can be let go of, it has to be painfully mourned. Finally, I will outline the importance of tolerating and mourning losses, and suggest that it is through the process of mourning that previously disowned elements of the self can be regained so that both self and objects can be seen more objectively.

Narcissistic Identifications

The more one studies these classic papers the more one is impressed with the importance of narcissism in impostors, who carry out their deceptions – sometimes for material gain, it is true – but chiefly to elicit admiration and seek aggrandisement. Narcissistic identifications at their most primitive involve a sense of 'being' the object in which no separateness between self or object is experienced. This was nicely put by Freud in a posthumously discovered snippet entitled 'Having and Being in Children'.

> Children like expressing an object-relation by an identification: 'I am the object.' 'Having' is the later of the two; after the loss of the object it relapses into 'being'. Example: the breast. 'The breast is a part of me, I am the breast.' Only later: 'I have it' – that is, 'I am not it'... (Freud, 1941, p. 299)

Greenacre understood this and described how 'The intense maternal attachment to which the future impostor is subject, as if he were a part of the mother, undermines his sense of a separate self and the development of his own identity' (1958, p. 369; 2011, p. 1034). Later, Rosenfeld (1971) described how a narcissistic identification defends against any experience of separateness and difference between self and object. It is the experience of separateness that allows the object to be observed as a whole and enables both good and bad elements to be recognised. Bad elements lead to frustration and good ones provoke envy, so that obliterating separateness is an efficient way of avoiding both.

In 'Mourning and Melancholia' (1917b), Freud described how the loss of the object is denied through the creation of an identification. The patient complains that he is ill, worthless, guilty, etc., and Freud recognised that these descriptions apply to the lost object. In the melancholic state the patient has incorporated a damaged, dying, or dead object and identified with it. Later, Klein (1935, 1940) in her papers on depression described how an idealised object is also internalised, alongside this depressed, persecuting object, represented by the maternal breast. This may enable a manic omnipotent phantasy to arise, involving the possession of an ideal object and leading to a blissful state such as that in the Garden of Eden. In a similar way, the father and his penis are internalised in both persecutory and idealised aspects. Deutsch and Greenacre describe how the impostor frequently identifies with a father who is omnipotently able to elicit endless admiration.

Alongside such introjective identifications, projective processes are simultaneously active and complicate the nature of identifications and object relations. In her papers on projective identification, Klein (1946, 1955) described how both good and bad parts of the self may be split off and attributed to objects. When combined with narcissistic identifications this leads to a narcissistic object relationship similar to that described by Freud in his Leonardo paper. Discussing Leonardo's relationship with his pupils, Freud writes

> The child's love for his mother cannot continue to develop consciously any further; it succumbs to repression. The boy represses his love for his mother: he puts himself in her place, identifies himself with her, and takes his own person as a model in whose likeness he chooses the new objects of his love. In this way he has become a homosexual. What he has in fact done is to slip back to auto-erotism: for the boys whom he

> now loves as he grows up are after all only substitutive figures and revivals of himself in childhood – boys whom he loves in the way in which his mother loved *him* when he was a child. He finds the objects of his love along the path of *narcissism* ... (Freud, 1910, p. 100)

Here an infantile part of the self is disowned, projected, and identified with the pupil, while the self is narcissistically identified with the mother. One could say that Leonardo adopts a false personality and in the process disowns infantile elements in himself. In this sense he is an impostor, claiming to offer maternal care while fail ng to acknowledge his own longing for precisely such care. In fact Freud observed that the pupil containing the projected self may become a sexual object:

> It has always been emphasized that [Leonardo] took only strikingly handsome boys and youths as pupils. He treated them with kindness and consideration, looked after them, and when they were ill nursed them himself, just as a mother nurses her children and just as his own mother might have tended him. As he had chosen them for their beauty and not for their talent, none of them ... became a painter of importance. (Freud, 1910, p. 102)

It is interesting that a completely different self emerged in those aspects of Leonardo's artistic and scientific work in which his capacity to observe reality was supremely present. In his artistic work Leonard seemed to find a creative identity, but when he tried to look after his apprentices' clothes, he falsely represented himself as an ideal mother. It seems that we can be both true and false in different situations as our needs come to be expressed or fail to be expressed. f analysis helps us to know ourselves, then it often faces us with the unhappy realisation that we are to varying degrees impostors, becoming caught up in projective identifications that defend us against reality.

When projection is used, excessively important elements of the self are lost and this may lead to a weakening of the ego, with the patient sometimes describing an emptiness and an inability to know what they believe. They may also be led to fill the internal vacuum left through excessive projections by internalising and identifying with powerful objects, both good and bad. The resulting identity may serve some of the purposes of successful living but is often felt to be fraudu ent, sometimes by the patient and often by others.

To make the total situation even more complex, we have to recognise that as well as being the active agent deploying identifications for defensive and aggressive purposes, the patient is also the passive recipient of projections from the objects they are in a relationship with (Williams, 1997). It is almost inevitable in our profession that we project disabled infantile sides of ourselves into our patients and narcissistically identify with omnipotent objects in an attempt to cure ourselves.

The Internal World

It is through these complex introjections and projections that an internal world is built up, which contains the self and objects in various states and in various types of relationship with each other. These internal objects are distorted through having elements of the self projected into them, and the self is to various degrees depleted by projection and augmented by narcissistic identifications. We still understand very little of how a sense of personal identity develops, but the idea of a true self uncontaminated by identifications is a schematic model, and in practice it is a fiction which can never be attained. All that we can do is to recognise some of the processes involved, and that when we move away from distorting identifications, we become a bit more ourselves and pretend less to be someone else. Nevertheless it is important to try to understand how such identifications may be recognised and reversed.

It is implicit in these descriptions that a true self can be postulated to exist; however, it is tricky to define, since it tends to involve abstract and idealised concepts like being true to oneself, being honest, and being genuine, all of which are rather difficult to measure and easily lend themselves to invidious comparisons. It is perhaps easier to consider the dishonesty and falseness of the impostor as a condition that we all find ourselves slipping into, and to ask how such a propensity can be understood. We can then consider that we move towards a truer identity as we relinquish identifications, and this can be linked to the idea that the aim of psychoanalysis can involve helping the patient recover parts of themselves formerly lost through projective identification (Steiner, 1996a).

Schematically, we can consider movements towards a true self and away from an impostor to involve a rediscovery of a self no longer distorted by projective and introjective identifications. Parts of the self attributed to objects have to be regained and recognised as belonging to the self, and narcissistically possessed objects have to be relinquished and recognised as belonging outside the self. Although always incomplete, moves towards this kind of recovery of the self can be observed clinically and are closely related to the process of mourning.

The problem is how to understand what might enable a patient to relinquish a narcissistic relationship and replace it with a dependent one, involving a separation between self and objects. While much remains poorly understood, this process has much in common with those that are observed in the mourning following a bereavement, and which have been extensively studied since Freud's original exploration of them in 'Mourning and Melancholia' (1917b).

Freud (1917b) describes how, following a bereavement, the first reaction is to deny the loss through an intensification of the identification with the object. If the patient can proceed no further, mourning has failed and the object remains concretely incorporated and identified with. The critical issue that decides whether the patient can proceed to the second stage of mourning is the patient's capacity to face the reality of the loss. In this second stage, Freud describes how

> Reality-testing has shown that the loved object no longer exists, and it proceeds to demand that all libido shall be withdrawn from its attachments to that object. (1917b, p. 244)
>
> Each single one of the memories and situations of expectancy which demonstrate the libido's attachment to the lost object is met by the verdict of reality that the object no longer exists; and the ego, confronted as it were with the question whether it shall share this fate, is persuaded by the sum of the narcissistic satisfactions it derives from being alive to sever its attachment to the object that has been abolished. (1917b, p. 255)

Today, as we recognise the central role of projective identification in the creation of pathological object relations, we can restate Freud's formulation in terms of detachment of parts of the self from the object rather than in terms of detachment of libido. It then becomes clear that as reality is applied to each of the memories of the lost object, what has to be faced is the painful recognition of what belongs to the object and what belongs to the self. It is through the detailed work of mourning that these differentiations are made; in the process the lost object is seen more realistically, and the previously disowned parts of the self are gradually acknowledged as belonging to the self. Some of these lost parts of the self are valuable and have been disowned for complex reasons, for example out of fear of being envied.

Others, such as aggression or rebelliousness, may have been seen as undesirable, but when regained are felt to strengthen the self. In any event, an enormous gain is derived from a sense of wholeness and integration. If separateness between self and object can be achieved, it has immense consequences and enables further development towards individual growth and responsibility and a sense of identity. Indeed, all aspects of mental life are affected, including thinking and symbol formation (Bion, 1962; Segal, 1957).

Moreover, what applies for the mourning connected with an actual bereavement is in its essentials also true for all experiences of separateness, which at a primitive level are felt as a loss. In analysis it is often actual separations, such as those that occur over weekends and holidays, which enable these processes to be studied, but the same process happens whenever the analyst is experienced as independent and separate and the patient has to face the reality of relinquishing possessive control over the analyst. If this can be achieved, a quantum of mourning can take place, and a quantum of self is returned to the ego. If the ego is strengthened, a benign cycle can then be established and a more flexible and reversible form of projective identification be deployed.

Problems of identity are central to the impostor. Deutsch's patient, after a good deal of analytic work, was able to articulate his failure to find an identity by asking his analyst 'Who am I? Can *you* tell me that?' – and seems to have realised his failure to internalise a self with a clear identity (Deutsch, 1955, p. 497). In the course of his childhood he seemed to have held onto objects through identification with them, and he could not tolerate losses and mourn them. It is also possible that his objects were unable to function as adequate containers for his anxieties, and in their attempts to relieve him, they colluded to encourage his omnipotence.

These two papers raise such fundamental questions, especially about identity and identification, that their richness remains fresh and allows us to explore these questions anew.

12 Personal Reminiscences from Interviews with Daniel Pick[1]

After some hesitation I have decided to include a personal account of my early life, in the hope that it might interest the reader and put my work in context. I have edited the transcripts of five interviews conducted by Daniel Pick in 2020 in the first year of the COVID-19 pandemic. I owe him a great debt, and his skill and sensitivity are evident in the text.

DP Can you tell us about your early years?

I was born in 1934 in Prague. The circumstances of our life changed dramatically when I was five, because of the war and the German invasion of Czechoslovakia. However, my leading anxieties had probably been well established before the war. Then the trauma of displacement to become a refugee must have been superimposed on the pre-existing conflicts. I did not understand much of what was going on around me, but something about my parents' anxiety and their urgent need to escape from Prague must have contributed to my own later anxieties.

It's quite interesting for me to try to imagine and to reconstruct what happened then. Prague was invaded in March 1939, and we were not able to leave until August. During that four- to five-month period, my father was going regularly to the visa office run by Nazi officials in order to get the required exit visas. So, I can imagine my parents being extremely anxious about things happening in Prague. I can actually remember hearing some shooting in the centre of the city.

When I was born, the political situation was already frightening, although I think it took my parents a little time to understand what was happening. The decision to leave Prague was based on my father's insight into the awfulness

1 Daniel Pick is a psychoanalyst and historian. He works in private practice in London, and is a training analyst of the British Psychoanalytical Society and professor emeritus at Birkbeck College. Publications include: *Brainwashed: A New History of Thought Control* (2022), *Psychoanalysis: A Very Short Introduction* (2015), and *The Pursuit of the Nazi Mind: Hitler, Hess, and the Analysts* (2012). He is also the co-editor of *Dreams and History: The Interpretation of Dreams from Ancient Greece to Modern Psychoanalysis* (2004).

DOI: 10.4324/9781003726135-13

of what was going on. Without his insistence it seems certain we would have died in Auschwitz as most of his family did, and I admire him enormously for his foresight. He went on a visit to Vienna around 1939 to my mother's family and he saw the way Jews were treated there. He mentioned a woman with a placard around her neck saying, 'I shopped in a Jewish shop' and saw Jews being forced to scrub the streets with toothbrushes. He was absolutely horrified and determined to do whatever he could to leave. Even at that time, my mother was not that convinced but he persuaded her. So, you can see that it was very late in the day that they realised just how vile this regime was and the danger facing Jews.

DP Can you tell us something about your parents and grandparents?

My father was born in a little village called Veselí nad Lužnicí, which is about two hours' drive south of Prague. It is in beautiful countryside with a big river running through the village. His mother was also Czech, born not far from Veselí, but she went with her family to Vienna early in her life. Prague and Vienna were part of the Austro-Hungarian Empire and travel between them was easy. She had three brothers; one was a postmaster and the other two were butchers, one kosher and the other not.

My father's father had six children with his first wife, four girls and two boys. When his first wife died, my grandmother was brought from Vienna for what must have been an arranged marriage. She inherited his six grown-up children, who were about her own age. So, you can imagine that she wasn't that popular, and my father was the only child of this second marriage.

My grandfather was a grain merchant and they had a large farmhouse where grain was stored in the attic and then sold on. They also had a shop that sold tobacco and groceries. So, the farmers would come with their grain and take back their shopping. This must have been quite a lively household with my father's six adult half-siblings. His older brother became a lawyer in Prague, but the tragedy was that they were all rounded up and sent to Auschwitz. One sister survived and together with her daughter later came to New Zealand, and another somehow escaped because he married a non-Jew. In the cemetery in Veselí, which we visited with my father, their grave is marked by a plaque with the names and ages of all the members of the family that died in Auschwitz, but interestingly, the plaque was positioned outside the churchyard because they were Jews. My father's mother was quite an educated person and would write letters for people in the village. She was not given permission to come with us to New Zealand because she had heart failure, and she spent the war in France hidden in a convent where her Jewishness was concealed. Having been a rather overweight woman, she was starved into becoming a thin old lady and her heart disease disappeared.

In 1947, after the war, my father managed to bring her to New Zealand, where she lived for about a year before dying of cancer. When we had to leave her in France, I was apparently extremely upset. We were very close, because while my mother went out to work she looked after us. Apparently, I wanted to stay with her rather than go with the family to New Zealand. When she reached us, I was 13 years old and I became fond of her, but could not link the frail little old lady she was then with the grandmother I had left in Europe. I knew her as Babushka and her loss is undoubtedly important in connection with my interest in mourning.

My mother was born in Krakow in a family of Jewish teachers at the local Yeshiva. I suspect that the men saw themselves as rather superior (I have photographs of them in their traditional Jewish garb). It was the women who not only brought up the children but earned their livelihood, which I think chiefly came from a corner shop that sold vodka and groceries. My mother's mother was quite a formidable, elegant woman, better educated than her husband, who worked as a draper at one point selling towels and shirts, door to door. When my mother was 13, they moved from Krakow to Vienna, and lived in the Leopoldstadt district, near the Prater fairground. She went to school there and then also to university in Vienna, where she studied physics, eventually taking a PhD. She particularly loved mathematics and when we got to New Zealand, she became a maths teacher. I remember her talking about mathematicians that she admired.

DP What are your memories of those five years in Prague, before the war?

I remember only a few incidents, but on a subsequent visit to Prague I found the flat where I was born in the new town, and also the one we moved to in a suburb of Prague when I was about two. It was a three-bedroomed flat, and my parents had one bedroom, my grandmother, my brother, and I had the second, and we had lodgers in the third. We had a nanny or maid called Lidushka who slept in the kitchen on a truckle bed, which she brought out when everyone else had gone to bed. That seemed to be completely normal at the time. She was an important member of the family and I remember being very fond of her. An early memory is of her holding me in her arms while we looked out of the window at my first experience of snow: I called it cotton wool and everybody laughed. I remain very sensitive to being laughed at, no doubt one of the reasons I'm interested in shame and humiliation now.

The language in our family was very mixed, and I think I must have been confused by it. My father spoke Czech, which was his mother tongue. He was 13 when his father died, and at that time he couldn't speak German properly. He needed to learn it because he was going to move to Vienna with his mother when she went to live near her brothers. My mother's mother tongue was Polish, and she also had to learn German when they moved to Vienna, and when she moved to Prague with my father she had to learn Czech, which she was never comfortable with. My father preferred Czech but they often spoke German together. In New Zealand they spoke English most of the time.

I went to a kindergarten when I was three and have an early frightening memory of two of the teachers, one dressed as St Nicholas with presents and the other as the devil with a birch. They came up to each child and asked if they had been good. Of course, I was totally convinced I was very bad and found it a terrifying ordeal.

When we arrived in New Zealand in 1940 when I was about six, I could speak nothing but Czech. Now, unfortunately, I can't speak a word of Czech, which is a great shame. My mother's parents lived in Vienna, and I remember one occasion when I was taken to the Prater fairground being very impressed by six elephants lined up a row. Children could feed them buns, which they picked up with their trunks.

DP How conscious were you as a child of being part of a Jewish family?

Not very much. In his adolescence my father was interested in Zionism, but they were never observant Jews, and later he became a communist and was always quite fiercely atheistic. In New Zealand, when I was 13, they thought it was important I should be conscious of being Jewish and persuaded me to learn Hebrew in order to do my bar mitzvah.

DP Visiting Prague later in your life, did it seem familiar?

Not terribly. There were a few memories of the flat and the garden where I played in a sandpit. I remember times that my father would take me out, presumably when my mother was occupied with my baby brother. I have a few quite fond memories of that, but also some frightening ones. I was a nervous child, and when my father took me swimming once he wanted to take me into the deep water, and I was terrified and refused. I also have a memory of a castle near Prague, about an hour away, called Karlstejn. It's a fairy-tale castle with turrets, and on a tour when we revisited Prague, I asked the guide to show us the well. The guide said there was no well, and I was quite desolate until we found an old woman sitting by a well, which was quite as memorable as I remember it being. She dropped some water down, and it took ages to get to the bottom. So, my memory was vindicated.

DP What were the economic circumstances like at that time for your family?

I think they were pretty hard up. To emigrate to New Zealand, they had to find landing money of a hundred pounds, and a friend in London borrowed it for them. My father was apprenticed to a carpenter, in the Zionist tradition of needing a trade to be useful in Israel, and when he stopped being a Zionist he decided he had better get himself a profession and became a mature student. It was then that he got some maths lessons from my mother, and that's how they met. Then after they married, they moved to Prague, and he went to Charles University to study law. They both worked for insurance companies, my father eventually in the legal department, and my mother with her mathematics was able to train as an actuary.

DP Do you have direct memories of the Nazi presence, and the immediate threat to the survival of your family in Prague?

Yes, I remember being scared, or perhaps more that my parents were scared. I remember an outing with my father's brother who had a car, and we were trapped in a roadblock and told that the Nazis were requisitioning cars. We were frightened but were not detained. There was a military barracks near our house and we had to walk past a German sentry at the gates. When we went out, my mother sidled me past the soldier with some anxiety. She was reluctant to leave Prague, suggesting, as many did, that a nation that produced Schubert, Mozart, and Beethoven can't be that bad, but my father was determined. They looked at 10–12 different countries as possible places to emigrate to, and since my mother's family had fled to America, that was top of the list. Apparently we were offered a visa to the US, but with a year's delay, which was too long.

The leader of my father's Zionist youth group was able to emigrate to New Zealand because his younger brother had been sent there as a young man. He was the black sheep of his family, and his father sent him to the most distant place he could find. This friend then helped us get to New Zealand. But first, we had to get out of Prague and to find somewhere to go while we waited for visas. When my father was 17 he saw an advertisement for Czech carpenters in France, and went with a group of 12 who were working in the tin mines at St. Brieuc in Brittany. He did various other jobs in the year that he spent there, including teaching Czech and German, and for a time in Lyon exchanged lessons with a woman called Germaine Goblot. They became friends and when we needed to leave Prague, he wrote to her. She managed to get us visas to France and even invited us to live in their house. She had what my parents called a Freudian lapsus and sent the visas for everyone except my mother. When she was told of her slip she quickly remedied it, but my mother always believed she had a soft spot for my father.

DP That must have been an extraordinarily difficult and fraught period.

I think it was the worst time for them. My father had to queue each week to see if an exit visa had been approved. I have my mother's passport which shows this visa with the stamp of the Nazi eagle and swastika on it. At that time Jews could leave, but soon after, permission was withheld. On the train to France the guards shouted at every stop, 'Juden raus', and all the Jews had to go and stand beside the train. My parents were frightened of a hitch of some kind which would prevent them getting back on board. Eventually when they crossed the border to France, they breathed a sigh of relief.

We lived in Lyon for around eight months, with Germaine Goblot and her elderly mother. They were an intellectual family with rather formal manners, and yet tolerated a family of five refugees in their house. They were remarkable people and later gave refuge to other Jewish families. But we were rather unhappy in Lyon. My parents had no money and no work so they depended on the generosity of the Goblots. After a time they found us too noisy, and they moved to stay with friends and left us in the possession of their house. I hated having to go to a neighbour to borrow a pushchair for my brother, and felt embarrassed that I could not speak French properly. I was actually sent to school for a day, but hated it so much that I ran away. The French kids mocked me because I wore Central European clothes with long woollen stockings.

DP Your parents were desperate to get a visa; did they realise they needed to leave France urgently because of the risk of invasion?

Well yes, it was early days in the war. It was 1939 and the beginning of 1940, but everyone knew that the Germans would soon invade France. We got a British ship that left from Southampton to Australia and we boarded it at Marseille. I remember we were already on the ship when they found an error on my parent's papers. I think my father had to prove that he had done military service in Czechoslovakia before we could leave. I remember my mother leaving us on the ship in the port and getting a train to Paris to get some document they needed. It was a terrifying time because the ship was only in port for a few days. Then the journey itself was a relief. We were all in one cabin and my parents would leave us to go to supper. One evening my brother woke up crying 'Hani, Hani', and the neighbour tried to help by finding some honey. In fact, he was calling my name since Hani is the diminutive of Hanuš, which is John in Czech. Recently I was actually able to find the ship's handwritten log, online, and this shows all of the ports we called at, with dates which correspond exactly to those on my mother's passport. We called at Bombay, where a snake charmer came on board, and a magician who made balls disappear from under cups. We went through the Suez Canal and changed vessels in Melbourne, arriving in New Zealand on 25th April 1940, shortly before German troops arrived in Paris.

DP Were you and your brother, four years younger than you, close?

No, I was rather jealous and hostile to the very idea of a brother. I remember I was even puzzled and bemused that my mother went to work. I didn't understand why mothers worked and had very primitive ideas of gender differences. My mother was always very independent, and my father was proud that his wife was a liberated woman. In Prague my mother organised the house while Lidushka and my grandmother did the shopping and the cooking, including providing for the lodgers.

I have a kind of double memory of my parents. On the one hand I remember them as extremely anxious parents, terribly worried, especially when I was a baby. I was fed by the clock, every four hours, according to a system devised by Truby King, a New Zealand psychiatrist whose methods were popular in Europe.

I think my mother suffered as she listened to me screaming between feeds, and I probably suffered a bit too from the strict regime. At the same time, they had a great zest for life. They took part in everything, they went to music concerts, they were very politically active, and had a wide range of friends that they invited to dinners and parties.

My father was a devoted communist until the Soviet political trials, especially that of the Hungarian foreign minister László Rajk, whom they knew slightly. Rajk was tortured and then executed and my father was horrified, and became vehemently anti-communist and later even right wing to a degree. In New Zealand there were lots of political arguments in the family, my brother and father usually siding together against my mother and me. Both my parents smoked like chimneys.

DP Do you remember your arrival in New Zealand?

I remember being met on the dockside and that we soon found a small house to rent in the middle of Wellington. I was sent to the local school and was put in a class of children who couldn't speak English. There was one other Jewish family we met on the boat but there were actually very few Jews in New Zealand. I think there were about 160 who attended the synagogue in Wellington, which of course my parents would never visit, but I was pressured to have a bar mitzvah. By the time my brother was 13 they had lost interest in the idea.

My parents loved New Zealand and felt liberated and grateful. Times were hard and I remember my mother noting every expense in a little notebook, but there was no unemployment. This meant that my father was able to find night work as well as his day job as a cabinetmaker. He was asked to veneer radio cabinets and since this skill was beyond him he was sacked, but with the typical kindness of New Zealanders they apologised and found him another job. My mother began as a house cleaner, but when her English improved worked as a teacher. They were very happy with their new lives, while I was more miserable, I think.

DP You began the discussion by saying that your anxiety is the thread.

Yes, I think anxiety rather than depression, although in adolescence I think I was depressed too. I think I felt something of an outsider and found it difficult to fit in. Eventually my parents moved to a slightly better house, which was still very humble, in a suburb near the beach called Island Bay. I spent all my out-of-school hours on the beach and at the surf club. It was a marvellous place, and gradually I began to feel more confident.

DP Were you hearing news of the war?

Yes. My parents felt a sort of survivor guilt and they were obsessed with the war in Europe. They would listen to every news item and follow every battle, sometimes with despair and then, when the allies were winning, with excitement. They also sent food parcels to Europe – mostly I think to Babushka, but also to various other friends in Prague and Lyon and elsewhere. I remember they would wrap and sew up these parcels in hessian cloth. They spent ages doing this, and I became fed up with all of this attention being given to Europe, which didn't interest me. I was a bit resentful, as if the war had been imposed on us against my will. I mixed with my New Zealand friends, who were more concerned with the surf club and rugby than the war. I did well at school, and I went to university when I was 17.

DP What was life like, in New Zealand?

Let me begin by saying something about my father and his situation. Having worked for a year or two on different jobs, mainly to do with cabinetmaking, he and his Polish partner, who was a very good tradesman, started up a business. They rented a small garage in Island Bay, near our house, and began making trays. They were extremely proud of the first batch of trays they made, which they stacked in a neat pile, only to return the next day to find them stuck together in one mass. They had not let the polish dry sufficiently and this first batch had to be thrown out. Fortunately, they had a sense of humour and were able to carry on.

My father was good at business, even though he disliked it and used to envy the craftsmen on the shop floor. Eventually they employed about half a dozen cabinetmakers, using a two-storey house where it was very difficult to carry furniture up and down the stairs. One day there was a fire and the house burnt down. The whole place was destroyed, and my father and his workers feared they would be unemployed. My father solved the situation by negotiating with the insurance company, and his cabinetmakers spent the next six months rebuilding the house.

Our family moved to a proper house, still in Island Bay, when I was about nine. And then, when I was at medical school, my father and an architect friend built a purpose-built house in a very lovely part of Wellington, with a view over native bush. So, they were becoming more affluent and comfortable.

My mother was a maths teacher and gained quite a reputation with her original teaching style. For example, she gave her class a recipe for a cake in grams, which they had to convert to pounds and ounces and bake. The class judged the homework on how the cake tasted.

In New Zealand you went to the local school. There was no selection and very little private education. My brother found school more difficult, and hated being compared to me by the teachers. He became anti-intellectual and, being keen on horses, decided he would be a farmer. His teachers said he didn't have a chance of getting into university, but at the last minute he changed his mind and my parents began a kind of pressure-cooker course of study with him, spending hours coaching him. He became determined to succeed, and against all predictions he got into university and followed me to medical school.

I went to university in Wellington for two years, preliminary to going to medical school in Dunedin. I joined the University Tramping Club, and loved walking weekends in the beautiful hills around Wellington. Then at medical school in Dunedin I made a new group of friends, sharing a room and then a house with friends that I mostly keep contact with. One of them, Alan Kerr, became a cardiac surgeon and another, Colwyn Trevarthen, who died last year, was well known to analysts because of his work with mothers and infants in Edinburgh.

I liked general medicine and at that time I thought I might become a virologist or a neurologist. In my teens I found a copy of Freud's 'Standard Edition' in the home of a friend and I borrowed some volumes, which made me curious about psychoanalysis. I think I was trying to understand some of my own problems, and it didn't take me very far. My mother knew a bit about Freud, having lived in Vienna in the 1920s, but I think she was temperamentally unsympathetic to psychoanalysis and later used to worry, perhaps with some reason, that mothers were blamed by psychoanalysts.

As I went on I became more interested in the brain and neurophysiology, and took a year off to do some research. We put micro-electrodes into the brains of cats and recorded action potentials that arose as a result of stretching a leg muscle. This was all under the direction of Professor Archie McIntyre, who was a lovely man and an excellent scientist. He became well known for his confrontations with another leading neurophysiologist, Jack Eccles, who had been his predecessor in Dunedin, over electrical or chemical transmission between neurones. In our research we showed that stretch receptors from the muscles send impulses up the spinal cord to the brain, in a bundle of fibres called Flechsig's tracts. I didn't know it at the time, but this was the same Flechsig who was Schreber's psychiatrist. About 30 years later I met somebody at a conference in the United States who surprised me, saying, 'You're not the Steiner of "Mark, McIntyre and Steiner" are you?' Unbeknown to me, the paper must have become important.

DP You have something in common with Freud in that respect … setting out from neurology?

Later on I thought that, but at the time I was turning to neuroscience because I was worried that psychoanalysis was not sufficiently scientific and that I might become duped into believing something pseudo-mystical or spiritual. So, I armed myself with as much scientific weaponry as I could to protect my rationality. I think I was always afraid of losing my sanity, and for example, I never took LSD or any hallucinogenic drugs for fear that I may not be able to return from the trip!

DP After qualifying in medicine, what did you envisage doing next?

I was already interested in psychoanalysis then. But here I have to mention another influence, Harold Bourne, who came to New Zealand from London and became a lecturer in the psychiatry department when I was a medical student in Dunedin. New Zealand psychiatry was conservative, orthodox, and boring, and he was like a breath of fresh air. He was rebellious and unorthodox and interested in psychoanalysis, having been in analysis in London. He collected a group of young admirers around him, and I was one of these, and very influenced by him. We discussed psychiatry and psychoanalysis but also literature and politics. He introduced me to authors such as Henry James, and all kinds of possibilities suddenly opened up for me. He gave three lectures on Freud, which were mind-boggling to me, because New Zealand was a place of down-to-earth farmers and rugby players and did not take easily to Freud. He was too eccentric to be accepted for training at the Institute here in London, but he had an original mind and seemed to show us that it was possible to rebel against orthodoxy. We remained friends when later he returned to London and set up a therapeutic community in a psychiatric hospital.

My main ambition when I finished medical school was to get out of New Zealand and go and see the world. It was a common ambition among young New Zealanders to go either to America or England. Harold and I were discussing what I might do, and I remember he said, 'Well the important thing is to go to a nice place–don't worry what you study.' He wrote a laudatory letter about me to Oliver Zangwill, who was the professor of experimental psychology at Cambridge, and this led to me being offered a place there.

However, just as I was preparing to leave New Zealand in 1959, Zangwill wrote suggesting I might delay my visit for a year, and I saw this as an opportunity to spend some time in the US. My old friend Colwyn Trevarthen was working at Caltech in Pasadena with the Nobel Prize–winning neuroscientist Roger Sperry, and he managed to arrange a post-doc fellowship for me. Sperry divided the corpus callosum of monkeys and showed that if you teach a problem to one half of a monkey's brain, the other half doesn't know it. These were called split-brain animals, and the work was later extended to humans by one of his team. I admired Sperry enormously but was rather overawed at Caltech, where there were seven Nobel Prize winners in the biology building alone, including Linus Pauling.

In my own research, I tried to use a split-brain monkey to make one half of a brain neurotic and keep the other half sane. Pavlov produced an experimental neurosis by training dogs to salivate when they saw a circle and to not salivate when they saw an ellipse. When they made the circles more elliptical, the dogs apparently became neurotic. I did something like that with half the brain and not the other half, but it didn't really work out.

DP Was the ethical question, about use of live animals, particularly monkeys, controversial in your world at that time?

Yes, it was, and you had to go to considerable trouble to get a licence and to justify the work. But I have to say, at a personal level, later I was horrified at what we did and I wouldn't go back to it. We used rhesus monkeys and over the years I developed a dislike of these animals, at least those kept in laboratory conditions. They are no doubt quite different in the wild, but in cages, and when being experimented on, they are vicious and awful. I was however rather insensitive at the time, and the same was true earlier at medical school when we dissected the human body in a huge room with 12 cadavers. Once later on, when I had qualified, I returned to this room and was so nauseated I had to leave. At the time we were hardened to it.

Later, in 1963, I spent a month in Warsaw visiting Professor Kornorski, who was a Pavlovian neuroscientist I had met in Cambridge. I was keen to see Pavlovian conditioning and I learned that the relationship between the dogs and the experimenters was quite important. Stroking the dogs, they would say, 'Come on Boris, salivate for Daddy.' The Poles hated the Russians and were very keen to impress them. One day an academician from Moscow was visiting, and Kornorski insisted that I should demonstrate the split brain work by cutting the corpus callosum of a cat. I tried to protest that this had to be done by a surgeon, but he insisted and I did open the skull and at least showed them where the corpus callosum was. I feel ashamed that I allowed him to bully me, and look back on those animal experiments with some embarrassment.

DP What was your experience of California and Caltech like?

I didn't like LA as a city. I shared a flat with my friend Colwyn Trevarthen in a large house owned by a Kodak executive, whose wife would make us lemonade by the swimming pool. It sounds idyllic, and was, except that the smog in 1959 in Los Angeles was unbearable; your eyes watered, and you had to go indoors and close the windows. I was a bit lonely, and my dating adventures weren't very successful. Colwyn married the daughter of the Kodak executive, and in the end I left for Cambridge, spending two months as an intern in a hospital in Boston on the way. I was very pleased to have this interlude in clinical medicine before going on to do another four years of research in Cambridge in January 1960.

DP Can you say something about your experience of Cambridge?

Cambridge was marvellous, but again I was a bit of a misfit. I came as an older student and I felt I rather wasted the opportunities there. I was at King's, but I mixed mainly with the postgraduate students. I shared a house with Bob Young, who later became a psychotherapist and founder of Free Association books, and with three other PhD students. One of them, Maurice Henry, was a brilliant mathematician and philosopher, who introduced me to seminars at the Philosophy of Science Department. I regret that I missed out on some of the rich culture available in Cambridge, such as the English lectures given by F. R. Leavis.

I had agreed to do monkey research with Larry Weisskranz, but chose to use intact animals without brain lesions. I wondered whether animals were interested in information alone, rather than information that led to a material gain. Did monkeys have something like pure curiosity? When you are at a bus stop nearly everyone looks in the direction of where the bus is coming from, even though, of course, that doesn't help the bus come any quicker. And that's what I set up with the monkeys, and I showed without any doubt that they were completely uninterested in information: they were only interested in peanuts. At that time, I was a bit of a Skinnerian – again, to my shame, but I admired the scientific rigour.

We were all traditional lefties in Cambridge; we marched to Aldermaston and our heroes were people like Mandela. Deborah and I were married in Cambridge in 1963, and we very much enjoyed living there. When I finished my research I was ready to go into psychiatry, and I was inching towards psychoanalysis. So, the next step was to go to the Maudsley Hospital.

DP How did you feel about moving to London?

They say that if you stay in England for more than three years you will never go back to New Zealand, and at this point I knew that I was not going back. The Maudsley was a very stimulating place. The professor was Aubrey Lewis, who had a reputation for intellectual severity; people were terrified of him. He was actually friendly and supportive once you got to know him. He was keen to make psychiatry scientific, and my background at Cambridge meant that I was viewed favourably and he supported me.

DP In 1967, what work environment and culture did you encounter when you moved to the Maudsley?

Intellectually the Maudsley was very lively. There was a journal club every Saturday morning; a variety of approaches were tolerated and the level of intellectual discussion was very high. The accent was on classification, with the idea that a correct diagnosis led to the correct treatment. All of the patients were on drugs and ECT was used quite frequently. I was sceptical of some of these treatments and the research which supported their efficacy.

It was a very enjoyable place to work, with a high standard of discussion. We thought the junior staff were much more talented than the senior staff, many of whom were conservative diehards, obsessed with diagnostic classification and viewing psychiatric illness as a brain disease. Aubrey Lewis, however, took an eclectic approach, and he wanted to have every branch of psychiatry represented at the Maudsley, including psychoanalysis. The important figure for me was Henri Rey, who was born in Mauritius, French speaking and excitable, and highly original. He was not interested in trying to conform or to curry favour or admiration. Aubrey Lewis had weekly 'grand rounds', where we would all sit in a large room and a patient would be brought in, examined, and discussed. Henri Rey would always say something highly unusual and unexpected. I remember one day there was a psychotic patient brought in who was completely silent to any questions. Eventually Henri got up and said: 'Tell me, for how many years have you been sentenced to stay silent in this prison?' And the man said, 'Seven years.' It was the only thing he said.

Henri was a complex person. His primary love was psychoanalysis, but he was also interested in physiology and biochemistry, and at the Maudsley he was very outspoken. Oddly, in the Psychoanalytic Society he was rather shy, and he didn't give a paper until he was near to retirement. He was in analysis with Herbert Rosenfeld, and although they respected each other, he was a great admirer of Hanna Segal. When I came to choose an analyst, I didn't know how to go about it. I asked Henri and he said, 'I'll ask Hanna Segal', and she had a vacancy, so I started with her. I think it was the best decision I made, but I found I had little basis on which to choose. I tried to do it rationally and I read Anna Freud, and Segal's introduction to Melanie Klein, without being able to make head or tail of it. So I decided to take Henri's advice because I knew him and what he said made sense. He was in supervision with Joan Riviere, who was famous for the severity of her comments. He told us how in response to his case presentation she complained that the material was jumbled and confused. Henri explained that it was the patient who was in a jumble; his other training case purred like a Rolls-Royce. To this Riviere replied that it was his job to make the material coherent.

DP Are you suggesting analysts might feel under pressure to tidy up the material when presenting it to the supervisor?

Well, that is always possible, but there is also a need to create order out of confused material. Henri Rey was not a compliant person. Apparently Riviere claimed that she had only two gifted supervisees, Henri Rey and Hanna Segal. Eventually he did give a couple of papers to the Society and was able to publish a book of his papers, but his writing was never very clear. He was much better as a teacher in person, where his supervision and seminars were wonderful. I used to sit in on consultations he did and learnt a great deal. We teased him because when he retired he built himself a little house on the Ile de Ré, and we used to visit him regularly there until he died.

DP Did particular encounters with patients at the Maudsley stay in your memory, and perhaps also influence the development of your thinking about borderline states and psychosis?

Yes. For a time I was a kind of understudy there to Sir Dennis Hill, who was the professor of psychiatry. His wife was a psychoanalyst and he tried to understand psychoanalysis, although not very successfully. I was a senior registrar, and when he retired, I became a consultant at the Maudsley. I had ten patients in a general psychiatry ward where we very much took a psychoanalytic approach. We developed an enthusiastic team and would try to understand the patient's deeper conflicts and anxieties. We also tried to provide personal care for each patient. For example, we saw our outpatients with the inpatients on the ward rather than in the outpatient department. So when a patient was discharged, he could return and continue with his group or individual treatment without interruption. About 75% of the patients were psychotic and in group therapy these patients were always lively, outspoken, and disorganised. By contrast, nothing ever seemed to happen in the neurotic group, who did not feel free to express their feelings openly. Once a week the whole team would meet in my office where I would supervise the two groups, and it was always very striking to see the comparison. It's as if the psychotic thinking made things much more available, although chaotic.

I was distressed by many of the patients, who suffered so terribly and for whom we could do relatively little.

DP Were you inspired in that work with groups by Bion's earlier experimental approach?

No, not really. I didn't know about Bion in those days and his approach was very different. Ours was rather pragmatic, trying to cope with crises and to keep patients from breaking down. Later of course I became interested in Bion in relation to groups I ran at the Tavi.

At the Maudsley I ran psychotherapy groups, and I learned a lot from all this. I remember being moved when a psychotic patient who had stopped attending came back and was asked by the members why she had been away. She said, 'I went away because I couldn't prevent the war in Lebanon'. It was a moving moment, even though it sounds crazy. I think she felt the helplessness we all shared about the state of her mind. The other thing I remember was that in one of these groups we had a very disruptive patient who dominated the sessions, and the whole group conspired to persuade him to leave. Soon after he left, the group collapsed, and it felt as if we had collaborated in a crime in ejecting an unwanted child from the family. We all felt guilty and hopeless. It made me remember that you must never get rid of awkward people. You need them in the family.

DP In the 1960s at the Maudsley, were you starting to write psychoanalytically as well as to think psychoanalytically?

Not yet, no. I was too junior and too inexperienced. I didn't really feel my way into analytic thinking until later, after my own analysis. I was very lucky that Aubrey Lewis backed me and persuaded me to apply for a fellowship, which allowed me to have a research job alongside clinical work as a psychiatrist. The research I did was on risk-taking and to some extent followed from my work with monkeys in Cambridge. Now I find it rather boring, especially compared to the richness of psychoanalysis.

I did some work with gamblers, but mostly I was trying to do experimental work, to judge how we evaluate risk. I did some research using game theory, the prisoner's dilemma for example. I looked at how individuals would choose between a cooperative move that involved risk, or a non-cooperative move that was safer. I published three or four papers at that time, but it's not a period I'm very proud of; it was, however, very convenient because I could make time to go to analysis. The atmosphere among the consultants at the hospital was hostile to analysis, so most people went to their sessions secretly. I am annoyed with myself that I followed suit, because I am sure that I could have openly admitted I was training. But I did not come out, as it were, until I had been made a consultant.

DP In 1967 you embarked on your own analysis, with Hanna Segal. What impression did she make at the start?

She was an unusual character, commonly smoking a cigar or a pipe, and she was very outspoken. Right at the start there was a snag because she said her fee was four guineas (in those days everybody charged in guineas), and I thought that was a lot. My friend Sandy Bourne had just stopped his analysis with Hanna Segal, and I assumed that I was going into his slot and would pay two guineas as he did. So, I was dismayed by the size of the fee, and her response was to tell me that Miss Joseph has a three-guinea vacancy. I duly went to see her, but I felt she didn't tune into where I was. I also went to see Don Meltzer, thinking I needed to meet a selection of analysts, but I think probably I was already attached to Hanna Segal.

At that time I applied for a grant that helped pay for the analysis and had an interview with Elliot Jaques. When I mentioned that I was having great trouble deciding who to go to for analysis, he thought I was crazy and that I would never get a chance like Hanna Segal again. So I decided to pay my four guineas and start. In retrospect I don't think four guineas was so outrageous, and the issue led me to recognise a mean streak in my character. I see it as an important defect, which makes me hold things in, rather than express them generously. In her lectures on technique Klein mentions that Freud once said that the worst patients to analyse are those that are mean.

DP Perhaps that links to what you said about your history, earlier on in this interview ... your parents' anxieties, about the potential loss of everything they had?

Perhaps, but I thought Hanna Segal was right to be more concerned with internal sources, and the rivalry with my brother was certainly one of them.

DP There was clearly something that drew you to her as an analyst. You had a choice and opted for her.

Yes. I think the most important reason was her straightforwardness. She wouldn't beat about the bush or pull her punches, but she was also extremely kind, and if I was in trouble, she was very supportive. I always felt that she was on my side even though she would not accept my nonsense.

She was also very forthright in her own views. She wasn't one of the analysts that try to be anonymous. She had the *New Statesman* in the waiting room and she went on CND marches, so all her patients knew what she stood for. She said that it's important to be neutral but not neutered, and I liked that very much.

At that time, and probably still now, analysts were not supposed to make their views known, especially for example on the choice of a supervisor. I remember flirting with the idea that I might go to Meltzer, and it was very clear Dr Segal wasn't keen on that. Eventually she said, 'What about Rosenfeld?' And I remember saying, 'Gosh, I hadn't thought that would be possible'. He seemed so high up in the hierarchy.

So, I went to him, and I thought that, at his best, he was the finest analyst clinically that I had met. He had a marvellous capacity to listen and tune into the patient.

DP You started your analysis in '67; did you very quickly become a candidate?

I think I had to wait 18 months or so. I remember being pretty arrogant and critical of the training, but on balance I thought it was pretty good and the supervisions I had were excellent, as too were many of the seminars. However we had small children then, and Deborah was always fed up with me going out to seminars in the evenings. Sometimes we were supposed to go to three seminars a week, and I found this too much and would miss some. I was always torn between the family and the training, and remember one day I got into the car to go to a seminar and drove two or three times around the block before deciding to stay at home.

Because I missed so many seminars, Pearl King, my progress advisor, summoned me for an interview. I explained my conflict, arrogantly adding that some of the seminars were not worth going to. I have to say she was very generous and said that I would have to make my own judgement about that. I had no further trouble and I assume that she stood up for me.

DP Did you have some sense of the effects of the controversial discussions and the divisions? Did it feel very fractured?

As onlookers, the students were rather excited when they got a glimpse of disagreements among senior figures. In the early 1970s we all went to the scientific meetings and listened to the controversies with excited interest. Most meetings were full and people were extremely outspoken.

DP That is what always strikes one about the 'Controversial Discussions' of the '40s: the acrimony and the high level of debate.

Yes. I agree. I thought it was very high-level stuff. I was quite admiring of the Society as a whole.

DP I asked you to identify some 'threads' that you felt ran throughout your life and you picked out anxiety; you spoke of your childhood and what you gleaned from your parents. Do you think there are particular threads of interest and concern running through your psychoanalytic writings?

I think the other area that I became interested in had to do with loss, and dealing with the capacity to tolerate loss. In particular, how it is through the process of mourning that a person regains parts of themself that had been disowned through projective identification. I have suggested that we could consider the aim of psychoanalysis not as a way to help people solve their life problems, but as a means to help them regain the capacities that were lost or paralysed, and it is in the process of mourning that parts of the self are regained.

Freud said, in his wonderful 'Mourning and Melancholia' paper, that in the work of mourning we take out each of our memories of the lost objects and apply the verdict of reality to it. I thought that, in this way, we assess whether this property belongs to me or to the object, and in the process of letting go of the object you can regain those parts that were projected.

The paranoid schizoid and the depressive positions can be thought of as a kind of equilibrium. Bion shows this in his famous diagram, which highlights that you move in both directions, forwards and back, but I always thought that he omitted something by presenting it as if it were a smooth movement to and fro. I was predominantly occupied with stuck states of mind, where a patient doesn't move anywhere. This can be thought of as a borderline situation, which at that time I linked with what Henri Rey said about borderline patients: they were not just patients on the border between neurosis and psychosis, but they seemed subjectively to feel themselves on the border of everything, as if they didn't know whether they were small or large, weak or strong, male or female. In every category you could think of they felt themselves to be on the border. I thought that these patients adopted a kind of identity which was borderline, neither one thing nor the other, and that they adopted a borderline position which was in an equilibrium with both the paranoid schizoid and the depressive positions.

Betty Joseph did not like the idea of another position, and she helped me to rename it a psychic retreat. If the depressive position was too painful you could withdraw into a retreat, and coming out of the retreat meant facing both the pain of depression and the anxiety of paranoia.

But I still think of a psychic retreat as a borderline position based on a pathological organisation of defences very close to Herbert Rosenfeld's idea of narcissistic organisations. Then another feature of a psychic retreat was that it appeared in the clinical material as a spatial concept, as a place, sometimes appearing in dreams or phantasies as an actual place to which the patient could withdraw.

I was very influenced at that time by Betty Joseph and attended her workshop for over 35 years. She managed to preside over a very high-level discussion between its participants, including Ron Britton, Michael Feldman, Priscilla Roth, and Ignês Sodré, and I greatly admired her devotion to the analytic task. She had a rather narrow focus perhaps, being interested in what was happening between patient and analyst, and nothing else. She insisted that you first had to understand what was happening and not why it was happening. This was a wonderful discipline, and I always felt that I was analysing in a more straightforward way after her seminar.

When I gave my first paper at the society I was very anxious, and I worried that I would let down my colleagues and teachers.

DP At what point, if ever, does an analyst need to give up the task of an analysis, or help the patient who seems stuck or unable to move to call it a day? Have you had cases where you felt the patient just cannot move?

Freud addressed this problem in 'Analysis Terminable and Interminable', where he suggested that a major obstacle to progress in analysis was the repudiation of femininity. I thought this was a very surprising conclusion and a highly significant one. I think he believed that both men and women prefer phallic power and fear feminine vulnerability. This meant that feminine qualities, especially receptive qualities, are felt to be inferior and repudiated by both men and women.

DP He was writing before the second wave of feminism in the 1960s.

Yes, and many feminists strongly objected to his ideas. I felt they misunderstood them, because Freud didn't think women were inferior but was describing a deep prejudice against women that he observed. This contributed to my interest in factors that prevent movement and lead to stuck analysis, and sometimes to interminable analysis. There are times when it is important to stop an analysis that's getting nowhere, and where indeed, it may be unethical to continue. While at other times there may be a blockage because of something we don't understand.

DP Many of Freud's great papers seem to be shadowed by the difficulty of the times he lived in, the experiences he had and evidence he gleaned in the consulting room. Do you think that's true of your own writing and psychoanalytic concerns? For instance, does your interest in psychic retreats or pathological organisations have a wider context?

Of course, the wider social context is important. The experience of being a refugee and the Nazi atrocities of the Holocaust all fit with an idea of a pathological organisation that imprisons the good element in society. Our recognition of the many good Germans who were helpless to prevent this organisation taking over makes us aware of our current helplessness in the face of the right-wing resurgence all around the world. Freud linked the destructiveness to the operation of the death instinct, but I think of the death instinct more as a clinical rather than a social idea. I think of it as an anti-life instinct rather than a death instinct. The life instinct gets weaker and weaker, and as I get older, I am conscious that death is much nearer each year and that the life force is weaker as I can't do the things I used to be able to do. This falling-off of capacities is intensely disturbing and involves the acceptance and mourning of loss. This means that our ambitions have to be relinquished and mourned, and we move towards our death having to give up capacities one by one.

DP Could you say something about what you did with the idea of the 'pathological organisation' in the mind?

The 'psychic retreat' took into account both the organisation and the spatial location. While the organisation could be externalised as a social system, Rosenfeld thought of it predominately as an organisation of internal objects. So, instead of objects being split into good and bad, and then integrated into whole objects partly good and bad, there was a fragmentation and a reorganisation into powerful systems. Normal family structure involves a hierarchical organisation that provides stability and allows development and growth because it provides security. However, if you are displaced from your place in the hierarchy it can involve a traumatic fall, which is felt to be unjust, and of course sometimes is actually unjust and leads to terrible humiliation because of the previously held superiority. Pride comes before a fall, and a high position in the hierarchy can be dangerous. Medieval philosophers referred to the hierarchy as the great chain of being, beginning with God and followed by nine orders of angels. Man was the head of the family, with women and children [lower down the hierarchy], followed by animals, and then stones and other concrete objects. I viewed a psychic retreat as an artificial organisation based on narcissism and omnipotent fantasies, which provided a spurious status which was very difficult to give up.

DP I wondered how important particular encounters with particular patients at the Maudsley and the Tavistock, or your private patients, proved in the development of your thinking and theories? I am interested here in how you feel theories informed your practice, but also how your practice led you to rethink the theories.

That would be very interesting, and I wish I could answer by looking at specific cases. One example from my experience at the Maudsley was the realisation that states of chaos, fragmentation, and confusion are often so difficult to bear that they give rise to delusional organisations as a means of creating order.

DP I think what you are saying here also connects to Freud's idea that in psychosis, the delusion may serve as a patch; it helps the patient construct something out of the chaos, so it's better to have a delusion than to be in total chaos.

Yes. When I began psychiatry it was still occasionally possible for patients to come into hospital without being drugged up to their eyeballs. Nowadays you rarely see a psychotic patient who isn't full of drugs. I remember seeing some patients who showed what used to be called a 'delusional mood', extremely anxious, feeling fragmented, looking around all the time, restless and unresponsive to others. Then by the next day they were much calmer and their fragmentation had become organised into a delusional system. They might complain that Martians were sending rays to poison their food, but the anxiety was confined to the specific delusion and not generalised as it had been before. The psychotic organisation gave rise to the delusion, which as Freud suggested can serve as a patch to hold the chaos in check.

Delusional organisations can also function as a defence against other anxieties, and I have been struck by how often humiliation is a factor in psychotic patients. Megalomanic delusions can create a sense of superiority by inflicting the humiliation on others. Schreber's account in his memoirs is a wonderful example. His illness began with severe depression and an inability to sleep, and his psychiatrist, the famous Professor Flechsig, reassured him that he would cure him through three weeks of sleep therapy. In his distress, Schreber believed the promises and his psychotic breakdown began when nothing changed and his hopes collapsed.

DP What led to your close interest in different forms of denial and disavowal, and your paper on 'turning a blind eye'? Can you say something about that?

I remember Pierre Turquet at the Tavistock telling me about a book that claimed that Oedipus did not kill his father and marry his mother in ignorance. He knew about his origins, who his father was, who he had killed, and who he had married. I then found the book, by Philip Vellacott, and was fascinated by his insight into unconscious knowledge and the mechanism of turning a blind eye. Vellacott was an eccentric classicist who taught at Dulwich College, and despite his many books and translations, was not taken seriously by the classical establishment. Later I met him and had several discussions about his ideas. He showed how it suited Oedipus to be blind to some obvious facts, which he and the people around decided not to investigate. I had a personal example when my Cambridge College termly bill had suddenly been halved and I turned a blind eye because it suited me. Some years later the college wrote, pointing out the error, and were surprisingly understanding and rather amused. Of course, if the bill had been doubled rather than halved I would have looked into it immediately. Normally an anomaly stimulates curiosity, but, as in this case, there are certain anomalies that are to one's advantage. The Oedipus complex is after all based on the fantasy of an ideal relationship with the mother to the exclusion of father and siblings, which is a very convenient solution to feeling small and dependent.

DP Let's go back to your collaborations. For many years you have co-run a regular event or conference, bringing together colleagues, mostly from abroad, at West Lodge. Can you say how that arose? And also something about your writing a paper together with Ron Britton that also became significant for many analysts – on 'selected facts' and 'over-valued ideas'?

The annual West Lodge Conference was started in 1995, first with Michael Feldman and Ron Britton, and more recently, when Ron retired, with Priscilla Roth. We had all been doing some teaching in Europe and the US, and Michael suggested an annual meeting at the West Lodge Hotel in North London. Invitations were confined to people from overseas so that we could present clinical material that was confidential.

It was a lovely setting, and the programme gave us enough time to discuss issues freely between ourselves and with the audience of 60 or so visitors. It meant that we each had to write a substantial paper at least once a year, and it is here that many of our ideas were developed and tried out in a friendly but critical atmosphere. Michael and I also used to meet regularly to discuss clinical work, and Ron and I went jogging on Sunday mornings, when we also discussed psychoanalysis. As in our joint paper, it was often unclear whose idea we were discussing, and we decided that once an idea had been mentioned on Hampstead Heath it became common property.

DP And your own workshops, at the Tavistock, and after? They had a particular format, a mix of reading and clinical material.

Yes, I always felt on surer ground if an idea was clinically based and not too theoretical. My seminar became known as the borderline workshop at the Tavistock, and has since been continued as a private postgraduate seminar. In the first hour of the seminar, a clinical case was presented and discussed, after which, in the second hour, we discussed some reading, which was linked to the case we had just heard.

DP Were you surprised when the book and the terms you used, including your actual title, *Psychic Retreats*, proved so influential?

I don't think I was aware of this. My interest shifted to the question of why it is so difficult to extricate yourself and to emerge from a psychic retreat. I became interested in the emotions that a person confronted in the process, when they lost the protection of the pathological organisation.

Much had been written about guilt but not much about shame, at least by Kleinian analysts. Of course, guilt is of primary importance and, without the acceptance of guilt, moves towards reparation are delayed and progress is held up. However, I found that shame sometimes has a kind of priority over guilt, and that the patients were often more preoccupied with embarrassment, shame, and humiliation, which had to be tolerated and worked through before guilt could be approached. As they came out of the protection of a psychic retreat, patients were no longer hidden, and felt themselves to be observed.

There's a wonderful passage in *Jane Eyre* where Jane's friend Helen is punished by being made to stand on a stool in the middle of her class in full view of everyone. Jane, who was observing this, said, 'Were I in her place, it seems to me I should wish the earth to open and swallow me up'. This sort of comment is quite common about shame, and indicates how unbearable it feels. It seems to inflict a trauma even though it does not involve any physical harm.

I came to the view that guilt is a deeper emotion and arises as a result of seeing your object more clearly, especially seeing the damage done to the object and, hence, feeling guilt. However, even prior to seeing you have to cope with being seen, and that means shame and humiliation, which has to be tolerated before you can face and tolerate guilt. While the patient wants to disappear and evade such feelings, the analyst can sometimes help them to tolerate and survive the shame. If we think of the fairy tale of the Emperor's new clothes, we can see that humiliation is a necessary consequence of the loss of the narcissistic delusion. You clothed yourself with illusions and are found to be naked. This is so often the psychological situation when a protective armour is removed; then you're naked and that's very embarrassing.

DP Or the illusory feeling the patient could have that the analyst is without or above such problems, perhaps because they are so thoroughly analysed?

Yes, some patients feel that, but there is also the danger that the analyst believes it and adopts a superior position. The patient lies on the couch at a lower level than the analyst in their chair, and it is the analyst who controls the time of the sessions, holiday dates, fees, etc.

A struggle over power and superiority may then become a feature of the analytic relationship, and it is here that an ironic stance can help us analysts to come down to earth and laugh at ourselves and our presumptions.

DP Do you think that your own way of working clinically has changed substantially over the years?

That's very hard to tell. I'm sure that in some ways I am less earnest and perhaps less therapeutically ambitious, but I suppose at a deeper level I'm the same person. People say I have mellowed and am not so prone to put people down. Sometimes when I look at my early work, I am pretty horrified, for example about getting into a power struggle with a patient or with a supervisee.

DP I remember you once saying in a workshop that a patient had said to you, 'Even if I was falling to my death, if I jumped off a building, you'd still be interpreting on my way down'? Are there situations where analysts are required to do something other than listen, contain, interpret etc.?

I thought this patient's comment was affectionate and ironic, mocking me for giving priority to understanding over action. However there are times when it is necessary to act, and if we accept that we have a duty of care towards the patient, it is sometimes necessary to intervene if there is a threat to the patient or to the setting. Sometimes I think it is necessary to put on a 'management hat' and stop analysing because of a threat to the process. But it is important to give priority to an 'analytic hat' whenever one can. In fact management is necessary to preserve the analytic setting, for example when we give the patient a bill. That is not an analytic gesture, it's a management gesture.

This means that it is not possible to get rid of memory and desire. I am sure Bion did not get rid of memory and desire in relation to his bills.

DP You've also said you feel there are situations where too much reality makes analytic interpretation impossible, and that the analyst should try to imagine it's a dream. That might free you from the reality – maybe a grim reality.

It was Bion's idea that sometimes there is too much reality for the analyst to be able to pick up the unconscious phantasy, for example, if the patient threatens suicide and the analyst sees the threat as real. Then he is so concerned to avoid a disaster that he is not open to the unconscious meaning of the act. Bion is said to have suggested a thought experiment in which the analyst sees the threat as a dream rather than as a reality. If he dreamed that he was going to kill himself, the analyst is liberated to analyse rather than manage the crisis.

DP As an analyst, looking back, what do you think ultimately has interested you most?

My writing has always begun with a clinical problem, and particularly with analyses that get stuck. Sometimes an analysis may make considerable progress, and then seems not to be moving again. I started thinking about this when I was at the Maudsley, partly influenced by Henri Rey's thinking about borderline states; not just borderline patients, but mental states in which the patient seems to be on the border of everything. Then psychic retreats became a way of looking at patients who were stuck. And it was important to understand what stops patients emerging from these retreats. They often seemed to emerge a little and then go back, like a snail who gets its tentacle touched.

I formulated the problem of emerging to involve both seeing and being seen. Seeing helps us to apprehend reality, including the damage we do, which can move us towards the depressive position. But the initial anxiety is more to do with being seen, as in the case of Adam and Eve, who were guilty but became ashamed when they felt themselves to be observed. It was this that first led to my interest in *Paradise Lost* with its vivid descriptions of shame and humiliation. About this time I had some discussions with Hanna Segal, who had developed the idea that the expulsion of Adam and Eve from Paradise, their so-called punishment, was nothing more than being forced to return to reality. The pathological thing was the Garden of Eden, in contrast to what happened after Adam and Eve were expelled, which was normal life. They were forced to face reality because their eyes were open, and with the new knowledge Paradise was exposed as an illusion. The Bible emphasises three elements of reality: the need to work; the need to suffer pain, especially the pain of childbirth; and thirdly, the most important bit of reality perhaps, was the reality of death itself. These three facts to do with work, procreation, and death are closely related to those chosen by Money-Kyrle as the facts of life.[2]

The idealisation that is essential to the idea of a Garden of Eden is one where time does not exist. There are no dead leaves and no green shoots in Eden. It is the timelessness that is shattered through the impact of reality that leads to the collapse of the illusion. The patient feels not only dethroned but betrayed, and the disillusion can be extremely traumatic. The loss is commonly felt as a descent into chaos and confusion, but is soon associated with feelings of humiliation that demand retaliation and revenge. It was Ignês Sodré who suggested that the chaos became organised into an up-and-down world in which feelings of inferiority and humiliation were followed by a triumphant reversal.

2 A person's initial dependence on the breast, the exclusion from the primal scene, and the inevitability of the passage of time and of death (Money-Kyrle, 1968).

Again, this is wonderfully portrayed by Milton through the fate of Lucifer, who had been God's favourite angel and was then unaccountably superseded by the begetting and introduction of Christ into Heaven. Like a new baby introduced into the family, this was a terrible blow for Lucifer, who became so enraged that he started a war in Heaven against God. Of course, it was a hopeless task, and he was eventually defeated and thrown headlong out of Heaven into Hell. When he landed, he was at first dazed and confused, but gradually he picked himself up and began to plan revenge against God by seducing man to disobedience.

In the infantile version, the child feels himself to be thrown out by the mother and, like Lucifer, he feels humiliated and betrayed. The immediate solution is then to reverse the humiliation by triumphing over the humiliator and thus creating the see-saw world of humiliation or triumph.

It is often felt that there is no way out unless the mother can save the day by reaching down and picking up the baby and somehow helping him to find a place in the family once more. This was Ignês' suggestion, and it means persuading the patient to give up his original illusion of being the sole recipient of his mother's love for one where there is enough love to go around for him too.

DP: This seems to take us back to the issue you touched on earlier: the patient has to come to terms with the loss of a dreamed-of paradise, and this might well include disillusionment about an idealised analysis (or analyst).

The patient's place in the family hierarchy can offer a sense of stability and safety when things are felt to be properly ordered, but if the patient feels unfairly discriminated against, the sense of betrayal can be aroused and the up-and-down world re-established. I have thought of this as a vertical orientation, which often uses anal mechanisms and phantasies. The patient longs to be back in a horizontal relationship at the same level as the mother, where he does not feel looked down upon.

DP Through all this current thought and work it seems you are revisiting in a new way Klein and the depressive position.

We could again consider the equilibrium between the paranoid schizoid and depressive positions. In the paranoid schizoid phase, with persecution dominating, the fear is of being destroyed, and shame is not so important when it is a matter of survival. In the depressive position, the guilt for destroying the good object predominates, but it is in the intermediate borderline position that shame and humiliation become primary. The function of humiliation seems to be connected with the establishment of one's place in the family hierarchy. While it may not threaten life itself, it is often a step towards something worse. In the Nazi treatment of Jews, humiliation played a significant part. The same is true of slavery, and the horrors of both these human tragedies involve humiliation as a means of maintaining the master–slave relationship.

DP Since you mentioned slavery, it brings to my mind how 'race' in classic psychoanalytic thinking has been an under-theorised area. For instance, how assumptions about whiteness and blackness may go largely unremarked. The assumption is of a white European male analyst, perhaps going back to Freud, and his, in certain ways, is a Eurocentric universe.

You have the issue of race, of antisemitism, of prejudice of all kinds; perhaps it is important to add prejudice against women and the hatred of things feminine. The basic mechanism seems to be to split off an unwanted part of the self and attribute it to another group. I have suggested this is what happens in the repudiation of femininity described by Freud. In the vertical-anal relationship that I described, anal phantasies are common and these come out when we project our bad elements onto women, or Jews, or black people, and speak of 'dirty Jews' or 'dirty blacks' to make us feel clean and superior in the vertical world.

The resultant power struggle was early on tackled by Freud in his concept of *Bemächtigungstrieb*, which was badly translated by Strachey as mastery. It has been revived by French analysts, whose work helps us understand the importance of reversing humiliation and gaining power. The anal quality adds the elements of control, and the demeaning of the object by dirtying it leads to feelings of disgust. Once you've contaminated your object and spoilt it, then you lift yourself with feelings of disgust towards it.

DP Characteristically, you use in your work powerful stories and suggestive metaphors, as did Freud; images or narratives that may have resonances for many or all of us – universal applicability. Do you think of there being a tension between that aspect of your thinking and differences you find in each case? I'm interested in how far you see recurrences and shared patterns, and to what degree you are surprised by the real differences that you find.

Interestingly, this is something that Klein spoke about in her lectures on technique, where according to Elizabeth Spillius she thought of two kinds of phantasies, the universal general ones and the individual personal ones. One can think of the Oedipus complex, the importance of envy and jealousy, and mechanisms such as splitting and idealisation that are universal. Then there are individual phantasies that refer to the particular experiences of the particular person who is the patient that the analyst is trying to understand. We could think of the individual phantasies as specific examples of the general ones. Klein thought that the general phantasies help to orient the analyst, but that it is the specific phantasies that need to be interpreted in order to carry conviction. It is too general to interpret that the patient is envious, for example; one must find a specific instance, hopefully one that is observable in the transference.

DP Just to return to something you touched on earlier, can you say a little more about how Freud's account of the life and death drives has been foundational to your own analytic thinking?

Yes, although I would formulate them differently. I think of the death drive as a clinical rather than a theoretical concept and try to observe the way it operates, chiefly in my view as an anti-life drive. It is mostly made manifest by the emergence of envy, but the idea helps us to understand that it is things to do with life and the creation of life that particularly provoke attacks. Of course, the death instinct and envy remain a mystery in relation to their evolutionary development. If envy is a hatred of life, why has it evolved? I think it is related to the mystery of evil, and calling it the death instinct or envy doesn't solve the mystery, it just gives it a name. We can recognise goodness and creativity in the world, and we can also recognise that a hatred of goodness and creativity emerges as a destructive force.

The laws of physics tell us that the physical world is running down, losing its structure and progressing relentlessly towards chaos. The only force moving in the direction of structure and meaning comes from biology, in which new forms are created. In the mental sphere we can think of the individual growing and developing from birth, but then with age we see a weakening of the life instinct as we move towards death. In the course of life, we have periods of creativity, but these provoke movement in the other direction, namely towards death. I think that is close to what Freud thought.

DP John, as we get towards the end of this set of interviews, I wanted to invite you to think aloud about your most recent work, and where you envisage it heading in future.

Recently I have been exploring what I refer to as the Garden of Eden Illusion and the consequences of disillusion. I became interested in Milton's *Paradise Lost*, at first because of my interest in shame and the meaning of seeing and being seen, but then the whole experience of the rebellion in Heaven and the expulsion from Paradise was fascinating. The Garden of Eden Illusion seems to be one of those universal phantasies in which a timeless bliss is imagined to have existed, usually at the breast, from which we feel we have been unjustly expelled. States of endless bliss are universally sought and we do not always recognise that they are based on ignorance. Once we eat of the tree of knowledge, we know about reality and can no longer believe in timeless bliss. We learn that all good things come to an end and that suffering and loss are part of life. In the illusion they are split off and relegated to Hell. The idealised phantasy is inevitably followed by the trauma of disillusion. For some of us the Garden of Eden is just a daydream, but for others it has a concrete existence and leads to what Akhtar has described as 'if-only' and 'some-day' fantasies: 'if only' we hadn't been expelled everything would still be blissful, and 'some day', Paradise will be restored.

Milton also describes the fascinating story of the fall of Lucifer, whose expulsion from Heaven leaves him dedicated to evil and revenge. Adam and Eve are able to find their way back to God by repenting and then making reparation, but Satan is unrepentant. Milton also allows us to make a distinction between the Garden of Eden as a concrete reality that can be held onto or regained, and a symbolic version in which the ideal stands for an aspiration or model of perfect goodness, but not one that can be actually achieved. Only when the actual ideal can be relinquished and mourned can the symbolic become its replacement. Klein had a similar view when she described the good breast as a symbol of goodness when it's no longer concretely possessed and controlled. This transition from concrete possession to relinquishment and symbol formation requires the work of mourning, as Freud spelt out in 'Mourning and Melancholia'.

DP That's right. There are many resonances to what you describe about some lost paradise: many variants exist in politics of utopias too. Your point about mourning or failed mourning could well be applied to explore past images of some state of 'perfect goodness' in religious and secular political visions.

We know that the only way you can achieve an ideal is to get rid of the bad by splitting and projection, so that Hell becomes a logical necessity if you believe in Heaven. In my reading of *Don Quixote* I was struck by how devoted he was to the recreation of the golden age. He was appalled by the cruelty of life and dedicated himself to protecting innocent maidens, while in his attempts to put things right he only made matters worse.

Both Cervantes and Milton deal with the issue of omnipotent fantasy, which is one of the ways a belief in the actual achievement of perfection is expressed. Satan persuades Eve that she can do anything God can do, and the Fall results from the impact of reality on these beliefs. However, Eve can be thought of as the first heroine who was able to rebel against the dictates of an authoritarian father. Sometimes omnipotent phantasies can help to extricate us from a subservient relationship that is blocking development. I explore this theme in a paper on the journey of the hero, where I suggest the hero has to embrace omnipotence in order to embark on heroic adventures, but then he also has to relinquish it, if his discoveries are to have a realistic benefit. Sometimes this is linked to the idea that anything new involves the overthrow of the old. Freud recognised that surpassing your father may be equivalent to a murder of the father, and that this may be necessary if progress is to be made. This means that guilt has to be tolerated as the price of development, and if it can be endured, the father can be relinquished as a concrete object and installed as a symbol.

DP There is also a question in analysis, that came to my mind as you were talking of works of literature, as to whether the analyst is perceived by a patient to be an independent-minded person who can think for themselves, or more like a servant of the profession, doing what they are told by others in authority. I'm interested in how much what you are describing through your stories you have also discerned in your clinical material.

Of course, the analytic setting is very conducive to a hierarchical relationship in which the analyst is viewed by the patient and often by himself as a figure of authority, leaving the patient feeling looked down on, criticised, and viewed as small, childlike, and dependent. If the analyst recognises his own infantile needs and conflicts, he is less likely to adopt a superior position and can be sensitive to the patient's discomfort and wish to stand up for himself. Becoming aware of his own vulnerability helps the analyst to take an ironic stance and recognise his shortcomings. Jonathan Lear (2014), in his discussions of irony, shows how often we compare ourselves with an ideal: for example when Kierkegaard asks, 'What is a Christian?', he means what is a real proper Christian. I found it interesting to ask, 'What is a psychoanalyst?' and hence 'to what extent am I a proper psychoanalyst'? I think the irony arises when I claim to be a psychoanalyst knowing I fall so far short of what I should be. We are able to aspire to something that we know is impossible to achieve. So that whenever we become a bit overconfident, we can enjoy an ironic smile of recognition of our pretensions.

My interest in theatre, and tragedy in particular, led me to compare analysis to the way we participate in the drama by identifying with the characters in a play, and then after we get home, or maybe in the interval, we step back and observe both the play and our involvement from the outside. I think it is this double view that creates an ironic stance. For example, in dramatic irony as exemplified by Oedipus, he and the other characters of the play are ignorant of the facts, while the audience has full knowledge of them. It is this gap between what the characters know and what the audience knows that creates dramatic irony.

When we listen to our patients, something similar happens. We project ourselves into their situation and empathise with them and go through their suffering and their pain. But, at the same time or perhaps later, we step back and observe, and this double reaction to our patients is both an empathic one and an observing one.

We are all like Oedipus, ignorant and then to some degree knowledgeable. And this kind of internal irony is especially prominent in Don Quixote. He is evidently quite deluded in his beliefs, and yet we feel a wonderful sympathy with him, even if we have to admit how mad he is when we step back and observe objectively.

Clinically, it is possible for the analyst to allow himself to empathically enter the patient's situation to understand his feelings, including his suffering, his mania, or whatever he is going through in a sympathetic way. But he must also be able to come out of that identification and observe from the outside.

A lot of this relates to this issue of omnipotence which we are perhaps too ready to disapprove of and do not usually empathise with. We tend to deny our own enjoyment of omnipotent phantasy and we can't then relinquish it if we don't know what we are giving up. Throughout history, omnipotence has been seen as a universal temptation and as a danger. The child inevitably wants to control and possess the breast and in this way to become equal to the father, and the only way this can happen is in omnipotent phantasy. There are countless warnings against hubris in Ovid's *Metamorphoses*, for example. Icarus flies too near the sun and Phaethon thinks he can equal his father and drives the chariot that carries the sun across the sky, leading to death and destruction.

It is this capacity to move in and out of identifications in a flexible way that I think is so important for a sympathetic analysis as opposed to a super-ego-like analysis. Of course, all these have risks attached to them: you can get a bit near to disclosure and over-intimacy if you overdo the empathic side, and you can get a kind of cold detachment if you overdo the observer side. It's this movement in and out that I'm particularly interested in, which I think involves a capacity for irony.

I think it is related to the capacity for symbol formation. If the analyst or the patient recognises that he has been thinking concretely, he can come to realise that this was omnipotent and relinquish the concreteness and move towards symbolising.

Of course there are some occasions, for example when anxiety is too great, where irony is not possible. The situation may be too real and too concrete for humour to be appropriate. It may then be too cruel to be ironic, for example, at somebody's funeral. Irony can also flip over into sarcasm, which is more sadistic, and there is always a bit of a superiority in irony, that you know something that the other person does not know.

DP When you have irony you may also have sarcasm, and mockery and derision – they all have different nuances.

Yes, and the effect they have has to do with whether you look down on someone or whether you have a kind of horizontal relationship with someone. If the analyst has himself experienced similar feelings, he is more able to speak at the same level as the patient. The patient and the analyst can then feel anxieties in common, such as happened when the Covid epidemic made everyone afraid that they or their parents or grandparents could become ill and die. They could then say, 'We're in the same boat.' At the same time, when the analyst withdraws and takes an objective view, they are clearly not in the same boat.

During the phantasies of the Garden of Eden Illusion, the infant feels in a horizontal relationship with the mouth and breast at the same level and takes this to mean he and the mother are physically and emotionally similar. He fails to recognise that it was his mother's arms that lifted and held him in that horizontal position, and when her attention strays he feels she has let go and he falls. With disillusion the Garden of Eden Illusion collapses, and this is always connected with a fall, often with a great sense of loss and betrayal.

Freud described an anthropological fantasy in which he saw the significance for man of adopting an upright position. Before that he thought of man on all fours, and like dogs sniffing each other's behinds when they met. With the upright position, vision developed a huge dominance over the more primitive senses of touch, smell, and taste, which require close physical contact. If we stand up we can look down on others and see them as dirty, and develop sensations of disgust towards them, and Freud thought that disgust was important in persuading man to adopt the upright position.

The early horizontal position between the infant and the mother is an illusion, because the infant is actually small and immature, but then when the fall comes he feels not just small but humiliated and betrayed. From his position at the bottom of the family hierarchy, he feels in a vertical relationship with the grown-ups, and his urgent need is to get relief from humiliation by reversing the relationship by adopting a superior position through omnipotent phantasy. This is what creates the up-and-down world where there are only two positions, triumph or humiliation.

DP You have spoken about the experience of the COVID-19 pandemic, and how patients and analysts might be faced with this common predicament; nobody is free of these anxieties and dilemmas. The analyst is not exempt. Particular historical and social experiences may bring shared human vulnerability to the fore. I wonder if this has echoes, given what you've said already about growing up in the '30s? Of course, that was a time when many analysts, like your own parents of course, were also at a loss, frightened, exiled, forced to become refugees, dispossessed entirely.

Yes. I often think that the present crisis at the height of the pandemic had elements in common with what my parents went through at the beginning of the war. There was a similar scepticism about how real the threat was, and now alongside the Covid crisis we see the rise of right-wing authoritarian regimes all over the world, including our own.

DP You spoke at the start of these interviews about your own beginnings, and fascism, Prague, flight, and all the anxiety for you of that time. And we are now talking about the pandemic again, our resourceful adaptations of work, the analyst's and patient's shared experience of this current existential anxiety.

We are greatly handicapped if anxiety is very great. We cannot properly attend to the patient and, it is difficult to use irony because the anxieties become too concrete. However, even then it is sometimes possible to be ironic as in the 'gallows humour' of the oppressed, for example when Freud could say that he could recommend the Gestapo to everyone. Sometimes, perhaps, if we are not too frightened of death we can take an ironic attitude, at least to ourselves, and adopt the double attitude in our work. Aristotle apparently said that the audience at a tragedy feels the two emotions of terror and pity. I see terror arise when we identify with the patient or the hero in a play and participate in his danger. Then when we withdraw and dis-identify, we observe his situation and feel pity. I think these feelings are important in the analytic setting. If we can't extricate ourselves, we can't feel pity and we are left only with terror. Sometimes it is like that with Zoom analysis, when we are so terrified of becoming ill and dying that we don't feel the loss of the personal contact. Remote analysis is convenient and a lot of meaningful things can happen and be understood, but it is not the same as analysis in person. Of course, the professional relationship in an analysis also demands abstinence, and personal and actual contact are symbolic rather than actual. In each case the gap between the ideal and the real can lead to the acceptance of loss and of difference. We can benefit from remote analysis, but need to take more trouble to compensate for the deficiencies it presents.

DP You were talking about the 'paradise lost' that people often have in their past, the stage at which it all went wrong. I don't have the sense from you that you're nostalgic about your early career in science and medicine in brain research, or have a sense of 'if only' you'd stuck with that?

Mostly, no. That wasn't paradise. That was me trying to be a detached observer without human empathy. But I am pleased that I continue to believe that it is the observing function that makes psychoanalysis at least partly scientific. But the subjective empathic quality is equally important.

Where it so often seems to go wrong is after the disillusion when paradise is lost. It seems very difficult to face this kind of loss, and we all dream of utopias of one kind or another. Mostly this stays at the fantasy level, but sometimes the disillusion is so traumatic and the fall so humiliating that the immediate need to deal with the humiliation leads to attempts to reverse it and reap revenge on the perpetrator. This means that the vertical orientation takes over and creates the up-and-down world of triumph or humiliation.

To relinquish the old and transfer libido to the new is a major task in development, and to let the old go we need to be convinced that it cannot be revived.

In this regard, an important step is to ensure our lost loves are mourned and our elders are buried, to witness them put under the ground – really face death, and the fact of the grave and the decomposing corpse. Until they are buried, the dead objects continue to influence the present and prevent development. This is the area of the destructive super-ego that it is so difficult to stand up to. Here, feelings of disgust help us to differentiate the living from the dead, both rotten food from healthy food, and creative ideas from dead ones.

DP It sounds like you might be revisiting Antigone?

Antigone insisted that her brother be buried to enable him to enter Hades, and this reinforced the importance of burial. It is related to the transformation of the concrete to the symbolic and the capacity to symbolise. Ashes to ashes and dust to dust, so the body is buried and the soul or spirit is released. In this way our mortality is acknowledged; we accept that the past is dead and buried and can only be preserved in the mind. When we see the dead, the evidence indicates the damage we have done and the violence of unconscious phantasy means that guilt is inevitable, because destructiveness is inevitable. If we can accept the guilt and not allow it to prevent us from moving on, we can learn to live with it, and with burial some of the suffering also comes to an end and we can bury the hatchet alongside the dead.

DP And here once more you are revisiting Freud on 'Mourning and Melancholia'.

It amazes me that Freud's paper, written in 1917, can still provide the definitive description of the work of mourning. He emphasises the need to accept the verdict of reality, and this includes the reality of our hatred. In Civilisation and Its Discontents, Freud quotes Heinrich Heine, who said that you do have to forgive your enemies but not until you've seen them hanged.

I think that is wonderfully ironic. It tells a truth, a cruel truth, that until you've murdered and buried the objects you hate, you can't develop. This process is counter-intuitive: we spend so much of our time trying to protect our objects and keep them alive, and avoid the difficult idea that we also wish them dead.

DP Often that late phase of work, whether it's art or in psychoanalytic writing, is the most poignant and sometimes the most profound. People talk of late Beethoven, like here we might talk of late Freud, as seen, say, in *Analysis Terminable and Interminable*.

At the end of her life Klein wrote a paper about loneliness, and she seems to suggest that when she was alone she felt that she had lost the good objects that had sustained her. This raises the question of what it is that sustains these objects when we are not alone. Internal sources of support such as the vertebral column can be thought of as an endoskeleton in contrast to the support provided by an exoskeleton. Initially we use the object as a container, a protective shield like the shell of a mollusc, but eventually, and it's a huge developmental step, the object is internalised and forms a backbone. We can recognise the huge evolutionary advantage of having an internal skeleton because you can take it round with you. If you use an external one you can't move freely. It is similar to Claude Bernard's idea of the *milieu intérieur*. When we lived in the sea we were surrounded by a saline fluid, and in a huge evolutionary step, a membrane evolved that enclosed a bit of the sea to create our internal environment that we can carry around with us.

I think this is the same in the psychological world. If you need external protection then you are bound to the external objects and cannot move freely. If you can internalise the object you can travel and develop and leave your actual objects behind.

DP I am very grateful, John, for this opportunity to record these interviews with you; and that you have been willing to spend all this time, thinking aloud about your life and work.

Well, there's nothing as interesting as yourself, is there?

References

Note: *Dates in the text refer to the original year of publication; page numbers and bibliographic details refer to the editions as listed.*

The Standard Edition of the Complete Psychological Works of Sigmund Freud, translated and edited by James Strachey (London: The Hogarth Press and The Institute of Psychoanalysis, 1953–1974), is hereafter abbreviated as SE.

Abraham, K. (1924). A Short Study of the Development of the Libido, Viewed in the Light of Mental Disorders. In *Selected Papers of Karl Abraham* (pp. 418–501). London: Hogarth Press, 1927.

Akhtar, S. (1996). 'Someday . . .' and 'If Only... ' Fantasies: Pathological Optimism and Inordinate Nostalgia as Related Forms of Idealization. *Journal of the American Psychoanalytic Association*, 44: 723–753.

Anderson, M. (2024). Entrenched Grievance as a Harbour for the Unmourned. *International Journal of Psychoanalysis*, 105: 153–168.

Bate, J., and E. Rasmussen (eds.) (2007). *William Shakespeare: Complete Works*. Houndmills: Macmillan.

Bion, W. R. (1956). Development of Schizophrenic Thought. *The International Journal of Psychoanalysis*, 37: 344–346. (Reprinted in *Second Thoughts* (pp. 36–42), London: Heinemann, 1967)

Bion, W. R. (1961). *Experiences in Groups and Other Papers*. London: Tavistock.

Bion, W. R. (1962). *Learning from Experience*. London: Heinemann.

Birksted-Breen, D. (1996). Phallus, Penis and Mental Space. *The International Journal of Psychoanalysis*, 77: 649–657.

Bloom, H. (1973). *The Anxiety of Influence*. New York: Norton.

Bloom, H. (1999). *Shakespeare: The Invention of the Human*. London: Fourth Estate.

Britton, R. (1998a). *Belief and Imagination: Explorations in Psychoanalysis*. London: Routledge.

Britton, R. (1998b). Publication Anxiety. In *Belief and Imagination* (pp. 197–210). London: Routledge.

Britton, R. (2018). Emancipation from the Super-Ego (Job). In *Sex, Death and the Super-Ego: Experiences in Psychoanalysis* (pp. 103–116). London: Routledge.

Butler, J. (1995). Melancholy Gender – Refused Identification. *Psychoanalytic Dialogues,* 5: 165–180.

Darwin, C. R. (1844). Letter to J. D. Hooker, 11 January 1844. Darwin Correspondence Project, Letter no. 729. Accessed 28 April 2022. lhttps://www.darwinproject.ac.uk/letter/?docId=letters/DCP-LETT-729.xml

Davies, R. (2018). Rivalry: Benign or Belligerent Sibling of Envy and Jealousy? A Clinical Reflection on the 'Winded, not Wounded' Experience in the Countertransference. *Psychoanalytic Quarterly*, 87: 265–285.

Denis, P. (1997). *Emprise et Satisfaction: Les deux formants de la pulsion*. Paris: Presses Universitaires de France.

Deutsch, H. (1925). The Psychology of Women in Relation to the Functions of Reproduction. *The International Journal of Psycho-analysis*, 6: 405–418.

Deutsch, H. (1938). Folie a Deux. *Psychoanalytic Quarterly*, 7: 307–318.

Deutsch, H. (1942). Some Forms of Emotional Disturbance and Their Relationship to Schizophrenia. *Psychoanalytic Quarterly*, 11, 301–321.

Deutsch, H. (1955). The Impostor – Contribution to Ego Psychology of a Type of Psychopath. *Psychoanalytic* Quarterly, 24: 483–505.

Dorey, R. (1986). The Relationship of Mastery. *The International Review of Psychoanalysis*, 13: 323–332.

English, C. (2023). *Melanie Klein's Narrative of an Adult Analysis*. London, New York: Routledge.

Feldman, M. (1992). Splitting and Projective Identification. In *Clinical Lectures on Klein and Bion*, ed. R. Anderson (pp. 74–88). London, New York: Routledge.

Feldman, M. (1993). The Dynamics of Reassurance. *The International Journal of Psychoanalysis*, 74: 275–285.

Feldman, M. (1994). Projective Identification in Phantasy and Enactment. *Psychoanalytic Inquiry*, 14: 423–440.

Feldman, M. (1997). Projective Identification: The Analyst's Involvement. *The International Journal of Psychoanalysis*, 78: 227–241.

Feldman, M. (2008). Grievance: The Underlying Oedipal Configuration. *The International Journal of Psychoanalysis*, 89: 743–758.

Finkelstein, S., and Weiss, H. (2022) *The Claustro-agoraphobic-Dilemma in Psychoanalysis: Fear of Madness*, ed. John Steiner. Oxford, New York: Routledge.

Freud, S. (1900a). Conquistador! Letter from Freud to Fliess, February 1, 1900. In *The Complete Letters of Sigmund Freud to Wilhelm Fliess*, 1887–1904 (pp. 397–398). Cambridge (Massachusetts) and London: The Belknap Press of Harvard University Press, 1985.

Freud, S. (1900b). The Interpretation of Dreams. In *The Standard Edition of the Complete Psychological Works of Sigmund Freud*, Vol. 5. London: The Hogarth Press and The Institute of Psychoanalysis.

Freud, S. (1905). Three Essays on the Theory of Sexuality. *SE* 7: 123–243.

Freud, S. (1908). Character and Anal Erotism. *SE* 9: 167–176.

Freud, S. (1910). Leonardo Da Vinci and a Memory of His Childhood. *SE* 11: 57–138.

Freud, S. (1913a). The Theme of the Three Caskets. *SE* 12: 289–302.

Freud, S. (1913b). Totem and Taboo: Some Points of Agreement between the Mental Lives of Savages and Neurotics. *SE* 13: vii–162.

Freud, S. (1914). On Narcissism: An Introduction. *SE* 14: 67–102.

Freud, S. (1917a). A Difficulty in the Path of Psycho-analysis. *SE* 17: 135–144.

Freud, S. (1917b). Mourning and Melancholia. *SE* 14: 237–258.

Freud, S. (1923). The Ego and the Id. *SE* 19: 1–66.

Freud, S. (1927). Fetishism. *SE* 21: 147–158.

Freud, S. (1930). Civilization and Its Discontents. *SE* 21: 57–146.

Freud, S. (1933). New Introductory Lectures on Psycho-analysis. *SE* 22: 1–182.

Freud, S. (1937). Analysis Terminable and Interminable. *SE* 23: 209–254.

Freud, S. (1940). An Outline of Psycho-Analysis. *SE* 23: 141–207.

Freud, S. (1938). Splitting of the Ego in the Process of Defence. *SE 23*: 271–278.

Freud, S. (1940). An Outline of Psycho-analysis. *SE* 23: 139–208.

Freud, S. (1941). Having and Being in Children, 12 July 1938. In *Findings, Ideas, Problems*. *SE* 23: 299–300.

Glover, N. (2009). Essentials of Kleinian Theory. In *Psychoanalytic Aesthetics: An Introduction to the British School* (pp. 29–64). London: Karnac Books for the Harris Meltzer Trust.

Greenacre, P. (1952). Conscience in the Psychopath. In *Trauma, Growth, and Personality* (p. 167). New York: W. W. Norton & Co.

Greenacre, P. (1958a). Early Physical Determinants in the Development of the Sense of Identity. *Journal of the American Psychoanalytic Association*, 6: 612–627.

Greenacre, P. (1958b). The Impostor. *Psychoanalytic Quarterly*, 27: 359–382.

Greenacre, P. (1958c). The Relation of the Impostor to the Artist. *Psychoanalytic Study of the Child*, 13: 521–540.

Greenacre, P. (2011). The Impostor. *Psychoanalytic Quarterly*, 80: 1025–1046.

Greenblatt, S. (2001). *Hamlet in Purgatory*. Princeton, NJ: Princeton University Press.

Grosskurth, P. (1986). *Melanie Klein: Her World and Her Work*. New York: Knopf.

Harari, Y. N. (2022). Why Vladimir Putin Has Already Lost This War. *Guardian Newspaper*, 28 February 2022.

Hoggett, P. (2018). Ressentiment and Grievance. *British Journal of Psychotherapy*, 34: 393–407.

Holmes, R. (2005). *Coleridge: Early Visions*. London: Harper Perennial.

Homer. (n.d.). *The Iliad*. (Trans. Richmond Lattimore. University of Chicago Press, 2011. Kindle Edition)

Joseph, B. (1975). The Patient Who Is Difficult to Reach. In *Tactics and Techniques in Psycho-analytic Therapy*, Vol. II, *Countertransference*, ed. P. L. Giovacchini. New York: Jason Aronson. (Reprinted in *Psychic Equilibrium and Psychic Change: Selected Papers of Betty Joseph*, eds. M. Feldman M. and E. Bott Spillius. London: Routledge, 1989)

Joseph, B. (1987). Projective Identification: Some Clinical Aspects. In J. Sandler (ed.), *Projection, Identification, Projective Identification* (London: Karnac Books). (Reprinted in *Psychic Equilibrium and Psychic Change: Selected Papers of Betty Joseph*, eds. M. Feldman and E. B. Spillius (pp. 168–180). East Sussex and New York: Routledge, 1989)

Joseph, B. (2003). Ethics and Enactment. *Psycho-analysis in Europe*, 57: 147–153.

Klein, M. (1929). Infantile Anxiety-Situations Reflected in a Work of Art and in the Creative Impulse. *The International Journal of Psychoanalysis*, 10: 436–443.

Klein, M. (1935). A Contribution to the Psychogenesis of Manic-Depressive States. *The International Journal of Psychoanalysis*, 16: 145–174. (Reprinted in *The Writings of Melanie Klein* (Vol. 1, pp. 262–289), London: The Hogarth Press, 1975)

Klein, M. (1936). Lecture 1: Guiding Principles. *The International Journal of Psychoanalysis*, 17. (Reprinted in *Lectures on Technique by Melanie Klein*, ed. J. Steiner (p. 37), Abingdon and New York: Routledge, 2017)

Klein, M. (1940). Mourning and Its Relation to Manic-Depressive States. *The International Journal of Psychoanalysis*, 21: 125–153. (Reprinted in *The Writings of Melanie Klein* (Vol. 1, pp. 344–369), London: The Hogarth Press, 1975)

Klein, M. (1946). Notes on Some Schizoid Mechanisms. *The International Journal of Psychoanalysis*, 27: 99–110. (Reprinted in *The Writings of Melanie Klein* (Vol. 3, pp. 1–24), London: The Hogarth Press, 1975)

Klein, M. (1952). Some Theoretical Conclusions Regarding the Emotional Life of the Infant. In *Developments in Psycho-analysis*, ed. J. Riviere. London: Hogarth Press. (Reprinted in *The Writings of Melanie Klein* (Vol. 3, pp. 61–93), London: Hogarth Press, 1975)

Klein, M. (1955). On Identification. In *New Directions in Psychoanalysis* (pp. 309–345). London: Hogarth Press. (Reprinted in *The Writings of Melanie Klein* (Vol. 3, pp. 141–175), London: Hogarth Press, 1975)

Klein, M. (1957). *Envy and Gratitude: A Study of Unconscious Sources*. London: Tavistock Publications. (Reprinted in *The Writings of Melanie* Klein (Vol. 3, pp. 176–235). London: Hogarth Press, 1975)

Klein, M. (1958). On the Development of Mental Functioning. *The International Journal of Psychoanalysis* 39: 84–90. (Reprinted in *The Writings of Melanie Klein* (Vol. 3, pp. 236–246), London: Hogarth Press, 1975)

Klein, M. (1959). Our Adult World and Its Roots in Infancy. *Human Relations,* 12(4): 291–303. (Reprinted in *The Writings of Melanie Klein* (Vol. 3, pp. 247–263), London: Hogarth Press, 1975)

Laplanche, J., and Pontalis, J. B. (1967). *Vocabularie de la Psychanalyse* (Paris: Presses universitaires de France. (Reprinted as *The Language of Psychoanalysis,* London: Hogarth Press, 1973)

Lear, J. (2014). *A Case for Irony* (Tanner Lectures on Human Values). Cambridge, MA: Harvard University Press.

Loewald, H. W. (1960). On the Therapeutic Action of Psycho-analysis. *The International Journal of Psychoanalysis,* 41: 16–33.

Mahler, M. S. (1972). On the First Three Subphases of the Separation-Individuation Process. *The International Journal of Psychoanalysis,* 53: 333–338.

Milton, J. (1674). *Paradise Lost*. Retrieved from *The Milton Reading Room*, ed. Thomas H. Luxon. https://milton.host.dartmouth.edu/reading_room/pl/book_1/text.shtml, accessed March 2008.

Mitchell, J. (2013). The Law of the Mother: Sibling Trauma and the Brotherhood of War. *Canadian Journal of Psychoanalysis,* 21: 145–159.

Mitchell, J. (2022). Why Siblings? Introducing the 'Sibling Trauma' and the 'Law of the Mother' on the 'Horizontal' Axis. *The Psychoanalytic Study of the Child,* 75 : 121–139.

Money-Kyrle, R. (1968). Cognitive Development. *The International Journal of Psychoanalysis,* 49: 691–698. (Reprinted in *The Collected Papers of Roger Money-Kyrle,* Glenlyon: Clunie Press, 1978)

Money-Kyrle, R. (1971). The Aim of Psychoanalysis. *The International Journal of* Psychoanalysis, 52, 103–106. (Reprinted in D. Meltzer (ed.), *The Collected Papers of Roger Money-Kyrle*, Glenlyon: Clunie Press, 1978)

Numa, S. (ed.) (2023). *On Being One's Self: Clinical Explorations in Identity from John Steiner's Workshop*. London: Routledge.

Ogden, T. (1979). On Projective Identification. *The International Journal of Psychoanalysis,* 60: 357–373.

Ogden, T. H. (2002). A New Reading of the Origins of Object-Relations Theory. *The International Journal of Psychoanalysis,* 83: 767–782.

Ovid. (n.d.). *Metamorphoses*. (Introduction by D. Feeney, trans. D. Raeburn, Penguin Classics, 2004)

Pope, Alexander. (1711). *An Essay on Criticism*. London.

Reisner, G. (2019). Ghosted and Ancestral Selves in Hamlet: Loewald's 'Present Life' and Winnicott's 'Potential Space' in Shakespeare's Play. *Journal of the American Psychoanalytic Association*, 67: 455–484.

Rey, H. (1994). *Universals of Psychoanalysis in the Treatment of Psychotic and Borderline States: Factors of Space-Time and Language*, ed. Jeanne Magnagna. London: Free Association Books.

Riviere, J. (1936). A Contribution to the Analysis of the Negative Therapeutic Reaction. *The International Journal of Psychoanalysis* 17: 304–320. (Reprinted in A. Hughes (ed.), *The Inner World and Joan Riviere: Collected Papers 1920–1958* (pp. 134–153), Karnac: London, 2018)

Rosenfeld, H. (1947). Analysis of a Schizophrenic State with Depersonalisation. *The International Journal of Psychoanalysis*, 28: 130–139. (Reprinted in *Psychotic States* (pp. 13–33), London: Hogarth Press, 1965)

Rosenfeld, H. (1971). A Clinical Approach to the Psychoanalytic Theory of the Life and Death Instincts: An Investigation into the Aggressive Aspects of Narcissism. *The International Journal of Psychoanalysis*, 52: 169–178. (Reprinted in Spillius E. Bott (1988) *Melanie Klein Today: Developments in Theory and Practice, Vol. 1, Mainly Theory*, London: Routledge, 1988, and in J. Steiner (ed.), *Rosenfeld in Retrospect: Essays on his Clinical Influence*, London: Routledge, 2008)

Rosenfeld, H. (1983). Primitive Object Relations. *The International Journal of Psychoanalysis*, 64: 261–267.

Sandler, J. (1987). The Concept of Projective Identification. In J. Sandler (ed.), *Projection, Identification, Projective Identification* (pp. 33–49). New York: International Universities Press.

Sandler, P. C. (1997). The Apprehension of Psychic Reality: Extensions of Bion's Theory of Alpha-Function. *The International Journal of Psychoanalysis*, 78: 43–52.

Segal, H. (1954). A Note on Schizoid Mechanisms Underlying Phobia Formation. *The International Journal of Psychoanalysis*, 35: 238–241.

Segal, H. (1957) Notes on Symbol Formation. *The International Journal of Psychoanalysis*, 38: 391–397. (Reprinted in *The Work of Hanna Segal* (pp. 49–65), New York, Jason Aronson, 1981)

Segal, H. (1993) On the Clinical Usefulness of the Concept of Death Instinct. *The International Journal of Psychoanalysis*, 74: 55–61.

Segal, H. (2001). Changing Models of the Mind. In C. Bronstein (ed.), *Kleinian Theory: A Contemporary Perspective* (pp. 157–164). London: Whurr.

Segal, H. (2007). Disillusionment: The Story of Adam and Eve and That of Lucifer. In *Yesterday, Today, and Tomorrow* (pp. 25–36). London: Routledge.

Shakespeare, W. (1596–1598). *The Merchant of Venice*. Project Gutenberg eBook #1515. Publication date November 1998. https://www.gutenberg.org/files/1515/1515-h/1515-h.htm

Shakespeare, W. (1600). *Henry IV, Part 1*. Project Gutenburg eBook #1516. Publication date November 1998. https://www.gutenberg.org/cache/epub/1516/pg1516-images.html

Shakespeare, W. (1601). *Hamlet*. Project Gutenberg eBook #1524. Publication date November 1998. https://www.gutenberg.org/files/1524/1524-h/1524-h.htm

Shakespeare, W. (1606). *King Lear*. Project Gutenberg eBook #1794. Publication date June 1999. https://www.gutenberg.org/cache/epub/1794/pg1794-images.html

Shapiro, J. S. (2005). *A Year In the Life of William Shakespeare: 1599*. New York: Harper Collins.
Sodré, I. (2004). Who's Who? Notes on Pathological Identifications. In E. Hargreaves and A. Varchevker (eds.), *In Pursuit of Psychic Change: The Betty Joseph Workshop* (pp. 53–65). London: Routledge.
Sodré, I. (2013). Death by Daydreaming, Madame Bovary. In *Imaginary Existences: A Psychoanalytic Exploration of Phantasy, Fiction, Dreams and Daydreams*, ed. P. Roth (p. 56–72). London: Routledge.
Springsteen, B., and B. Obama (2021). Relationships with Our Fathers and Masculinity. *Renegades: Born in the USA*. Podcast audio. 24 May 2021. 33:52. https://podcasts.apple.com/us/podcast/renegades-born-in-the-usa/id1562920267
Steiner, J. (1993a). *Psychic Retreats: Pathological Organisations of the Personality in Psychotic, Neurotic and Borderline Patients*. London, New York: Routledge.
Steiner, J. (1993b). The Recovery of Parts of the Self Lost through Projective Identification: The Role of Mourning. In *Psychic Retreats: Pathological Organisations of the Personality in Psychotic, Neurotic and Borderline Patients* (pp. 54–63). London, New York: Routledge.
Steiner, J. (1996a). The Aim of Psychoanalysis in Theory and in Practice. *The International Journal of Psychoanalysis, 77*, 1073–1083.
Steiner, J. (1996b). Revenge and Resentment in the 'Oedipus Situation'. *The International Journal of Psychoanalysis, 77*, 433–443.
Steiner, J. (1999). The Struggle for Dominance in the Oedipus Situation. *Canadian Journal of Psychoanalysis, 7*: 161–177.
Steiner, J. (2005). The Conflict between Mourning and Melancholia. *Psychoanalytic Quarterly*, 74, 83–104. (Reprinted in *Seeing and Being Seen: Emerging from a Psychic Retreat* (pp. 149–166). London, New York: Routledge, 2011)
Steiner, J. (2006). Interpretative Enactments and the Analytic Setting. *The International Journal of* Psychoanalysis, 87: 315–320.
Steiner, J. (2011a). Seeing *and Being Seen: Emerging from a Psychic Retreat.* London, New York: Routledge.
Steiner, J. (2011b). The Numbing Feeling of Reality. *Psychoanalytic Quarterly*, 80: 73–89.
Steiner, J. (2011c). The Impostor Revisited. *Psychoanalytic Quarterly*, 80: 1061–1071.
Steiner, J. (2015). Seeing and Being Seen: Shame in the Clinical Situation. *The International Journal of Psychoanalysis*, 96: 1589–1601.
Steiner, J. (2017). *Lectures on Technique by Melanie Klein: Edited with Critical Review by John Steiner*, ed. J. Steiner. London, New York: Routledge.
Steiner, J. (2018). Time and the Garden of Eden Illusion. *The International Journal of Psychoanalysis*, 99 : 1274–1287.
Steiner, J. (2020). The Sympathetic Imagination: Keats and the Movement In and Out of Projective Identification. In *Illusion, Disillusion, and Irony in Psychoanalysis* (pp. 101–115). London, New York: Routledge.
Steiner, J. (2023a). Foreword. In S. Numa (ed.), *On Being One's Self: Clinical Explorations in Identity from John Steiner's Workshop* (pp. xiv–xx). London, New York: Routledge.
Steiner, J. (2023b). A Kleinian Appreciation of the Ego and the Id (1923–2023). *The International Journal of Psychoanalysis*, 104: 1110–1120.
Steiner, J. (2023c). Mourning in Hamlet: Turning Ancestral Ghosts into Ancestors. *The International Journal of Psychoanalysis*, 104: 1025–1041.

Steiner, J. (2024). Differentiating Between Romantic and Mature Love: Revisiting the Three Caskets. *The International Journal of Psychoanalysis*, 105: 564–575.
Steiner, J. (2025a). Injury, Grievance, and Revenge, in the Wrath of Achilles. *The International Journal of Psychoanalysis*, 106: 784–798.
Steiner, J. (2025b). Before and After the Fall: Horizontal and Vertical Object Orientations in the Analysis of a Patient with Grievances. *The International Journal of Psychoanalysis*, 106: 873–891.
Stoller, R. (1975). Pornography and Perversion. In *Perversion: The Erotic Form of Hatred* (pp. 64–91). Brighton: Harvester Press.
Strachey, J. (1934). The Nature of the Therapeutic Action of Psycho-analysis. *The International Journal of Psychoanalysis*, 15: 127–159. (Reprinted in *The International Journal of* Psychoanalysis, 50: 275–295 (1969)).
Tennyson, A. (1850). *In Memoriam A. H. H.* London: Edward Moxon. (Project Gutenberg eBook #70950. Publication date June 2023. https://www.gutenberg.org/cache/epub/70950/pg70950-images.html
Tóibín, C. (2015). *On Elizabeth Bishop*. Princeton, NJ: Princeton University Press.
Weiss, H. (2008). Romantic Perversion: The Role of Envy in the Creation of a Timeless Universe. In P. Roth and A. Lemma (eds.), *Envy and Gratitude Revisited* (pp. 152–167). London: International Psychoanalytic Association.
Weiss, H. (2020). A River with Several Different Tributary Streams: Reflections on the Repetition Compulsion. *The International Journal of Psychoanalysis*, 101: 1172–1187.
Wilde, O. (1899). *The Importance of Being Earnest*. London: Leonard Smithers & Co. Project Gutenberg eBook #844. https://www.gutenberg.org/files/844/844-h/844-h.htm.
Williams, G. (1997). Reflections on Some Dynamics of Eating Disorders: 'No Entry' Defences and Foreign Bodies. *The International Journal of Psychoanalysis*, 78: 927–941.
Winnicott, D. W. (1965). *The Maturational Processes and the Facilitating Environment: Studies in the Theory of Emotional Development*. London: The Hogarth Press and the Institute of Psycho-Analysis.
Winnicott, D. W. (1974). Fear of Breakdown. *International Review of Psychoanalysis* 1: 103–107.
Wurmser, L. (2009). The Superego as the Herald of Resentment. *Psychoanalytic Inquiry*, 29(5): 386–410.

Index